100 Questions & Answers About Caring for Family or Friends with Cancer

DATE DUE

S

Me

Ri

Me

World Headquarters
Jones and Bartlett
Publishers
40 Tall Pine Drive
Sudbury, MA 01776
info@jbpub.com
www.jbpub.com

Jones and Bartlett
Publishers Canada
2406 Nikanna Road
Mississauga, ON L5C 2W6
CANADA

Jones and Bartlett
Publishers International
Barb House, Barb Mews
London W6 7PA
UK

The authors, editors, and publisher have made every effort to provide accurate information.
However, they are not responsible for errors, omissions, or for any outcomes related to the use
of the contents of this book and take no responsibility for the use of any products described
herein. Treatments and side effects described in this book may not be applicable to all patients;
likewise, some patients may require a dose or experience a side effect that is not described
herein. The reader should confer with his or her own physician regarding specific treatments
and side effects. Comments from a patient or patients used in this text are the opinions of the
commenter and should not be construed as representative of the authors' or publisher's view-
point.

Library of Congress Cataloging-in-Publication Data

Rose, Susannah.
  100 questions & answers about caring for family or friends with cancer /
Susannah L. Rose, Richard Hara.-- 1st ed.
    p. cm.
  Includes index.
  ISBN 0-7637-2361-4 (pbk.)
  1. Cancer--Palliative treatment. 2. Cancer--Home care. 3. Caregivers.
I. Title: 100 questions and answers about caring for family or friends with
cancer. II. Title: One hundred questions & answers about caring for family
or friends with cancer. III. Title: One hundred questions and answers about
caring for family or friends with cancer. IV. Hara, Richard. V. Title.
  RC271.P33R67 2005
  616.99'406--dc22

                                                                2004008516

Production Credits
Chief Executive Officer: Clayton Jones
Chief Operating Officer: Don W. Jones, Jr.
President, Higher Education and Professional Publishing: Robert W. Holland, Jr.
V.P., Sales and Marketing: William J. Kane
V.P., Design and Production: Anne Spencer
V.P., Manufacturing and Inventory Control: Therese Bräuer
Executive Publisher: Christopher Davis
Special Projects Editor: Elizabeth Platt
Editorial Assistant: Kathy Richardson
Text Design: Kristin Ohlin
Cover Design: Philip Regan
Composition: Northeast Compositors, Inc.
Text and Cover Printing: Malloy, Inc.

Printed in the United States of America
08 07 06 05 04   10 9 8 7 6 5 4 3 2 1

Brush Above Juneau

Fell off the trail
To Granite Basin today
Going through a berry thicket.
Brush up to my neck
All of the sudden
Like wading a creek
And dropping right into
A deep hole.
I disappeared,
Caught my breath
And some branches,
Noticed some little blue
Flowers low down
Before I bobbed
To the top
And kept going.

By Howard McCord

Contents

Estimates vary, but there are up to 9 million cancer survivors in the United States. In fact, you probably know a person with cancer: maybe it is a friend, a coworker or a former classmate. Or, perhaps it is someone closer, such as a parent or spouse. Perhaps it is you.

What was your reaction when you first heard that someone you knew was diagnosed with cancer? Beyond the initial shock and the fear, the feeling most people have is uncertainty. This is because cancer is not simply a physical disorder of the body: It is an idea or symbol that can represent and express our deepest fears about life and potential loss. Cancer still evokes dread in most people despite decades of public education and the tireless efforts of advocates to reshape previous notions of cancer as a death sentence that stigmatized and isolated people with cancer. Although cancer is common in modern societies, it is still not something most people normally talk about in their everyday lives.

Our primary responsibility as social workers at an oncology research hospital is to provide counseling to people with cancer and their family members. Through our thousands of conversations with the loved ones of cancer patients, we have found that this disease profoundly touches the entire family. Just as the people with cancer adjust to the news of their diagnosis, those close to them also experience their own thoughts, emotions, and concerns. If you are someone close to a person with cancer, this book will address many of the questions you may have. This book is intended to focus on the unique issues family and friends face when a loved one has cancer. By family, we mean anyone a person considers to be part of his or her "family," which can include blood relatives, a partner/spouse, or other people close to the person with cancer or caregivers. Some people consider their closest friend to be part of their family, while others consider only their spouse and children or their family of origin to be "family."

You can read this book chronologically or skip to questions that currently interest you the most. Some questions specify "my spouse" or "my partner" or "my mother." We used these terms simply for style and to make the questions easier to read, but in most cases the content applies to any family or friendship relationship with the patient. So, even if you are a brother or friend of a person with cancer, and the question is written from the perspective of a spouse, the information could still be important to you. We also use the terms "patient," "loved one," or "person with cancer" interchangeably. Our intention is to provide accurate, practical information and advice about common questions that may arise.

In this book we will provide you with major principles and straightforward tips to follow in order to support and care for the person with cancer, as well as yourself. Keep in mind, though, that people—and cancer experiences—come in all shapes and sizes. What's right for you may not work for someone else, and vice versa. Despite the diversity of experiences, we have heard numerous recurring themes that often arise in the form of questions in our work of counseling patients and their friends and family. The broad sampling of questions we have chosen for this book is meant to capture both the general and specific questions that might occur. We explore how to:

- Provide emotional support to the patient/other family and friends
- Locate support groups and counseling
- Communicate with doctors and other medical staff
- Research medical aspects of the disease from books, the Internet or other sources
- Serve as a point-person for questions from family, friends, and other people
- Care for a person at home, including sometimes learning new skills

- Negotiate with insurance companies and begin financial planning

This first section covers some basic territory—what cancer is and how you communicate with and generally support a person with cancer. For readers more deeply involved with the person with cancer or in providing care, this section is the foundation for successfully navigating and negotiating the issues that may arise later.

We thank the many people involved in the completion of this book, including Jennifer and Howard McCord, Jenna Daly, Widney Brown, JD, and Robert Wittes, MD, for reviewing the manuscript. We also thank our spouses and families for their support and encouragement, not only during the writing of this book, but also in the work that we do with people with cancer and their families. We extend our appreciation to our colleagues and Jane Bowling, DSW for her professional mentorship. In particular, we would like to remember all the people with cancer and their loved ones whom we have encountered during our years at Memorial Sloan-Kettering Cancer Center. Their stories and strength are a continuing inspiration to us.

Susannah L. Rose, MSSW
Richard Hara, PhD, MSSW

Publisher's Acknowledgment: Selected questions in this book include commentary by two people with experience caring for cancer patients. Mark T. Hamblin was primary caregiver for his mother during her battles with colon and breast cancer, and he currently offers support and assistance to two friends undergoing cancer treatment. The Rev. Canon Nancy Van Dyke Platt, herself a cancer survivor, is trained in pastoral care of terminally ill cancer patients and has assisted in caring for her own family members with cancer. We thank them for offering their experiences to the readers of this book.

PART ONE

The Basics

What is cancer? How is it treated?

How do I offer to help a person with cancer?

What does it mean to be a "caregiver"?

More . . .

1. What is cancer?

When people hear the word cancer, they think of it as some "thing" in the body: a lump, a mass—the tumor. Look in a medical textbook, however, and you will find cancer defined as an abnormal and uncontrolled growth of cells—a process. To understand how these two are connected, we first need to understand some basic biology.

The human body is made up of different parts, called organs, each performing a particular job that contributes to the functioning of the body as a whole: For example, the lungs bring oxygen to our blood and take away carbon dioxide, while the heart pumps the blood through the body. These organs, and other kinds of tissue that make up the parts of the body, are likewise made up of smaller units, called cells. Normally, cells divide and mature, performing jobs that are programmed into their genes, until they age and die, usually to be replaced by new cells.

A cell turns cancerous when something goes wrong in this process of cell division. A mutation alters one or more of a cell's genes; the cell then starts to divide more rapidly than is normal, and the resulting cells fail to develop and perform properly. While normal cells have as part of their genetic programming instructions to die and to make way for new cells, cancer cells do not have this mechanism and continue to grow unchecked. They accumulate to form a mass, or tumor, and then invade the normal tissue surrounding them, impairing or destroying its ability to function as well. Cancer cells can also spread, or metastasize, to other organs and areas of the body where this process of unchecked growth and harm is repeated.

Depending on where it originates, cancer tends to grow and spread in characteristic ways. On the one hand, this makes it possible to define specific guidelines for the diagnosis, cancer **staging**, and treatment for each kind of cancer. But because of these differences, cancer is in reality over 200 different diseases. Although medical science has grasped the basic biology underlying cancer as a process, the exact mechanisms for each type of cancer remain to be worked out. A number of factors can initiate the process of creating a **malignancy**: exposure to chemical and industrial compounds in the environment; medical drugs, such as some hormonal and immunosuppressive agents; radiation exposure; and lifestyle factors, particularly tobacco and alcohol consumption.

Carcinogens are those agents that directly cause cells to grow in an abnormal manner, for example, by altering a cell's **DNA**. There are also cancer promoters and enhancers that either create conditions that contribute to cancer development or accelerate the abnormal growth of cells. Cancer development is a multistage process, and it takes a number of things to go wrong in order for the disease to take root and grow. That is why not everyone who smokes will develop lung cancer, even though there is no question of the carcinogenic potential of many of the chemical compounds contained in tobacco smoke.

When your loved one is diagnosed with cancer, it is natural to wonder: Why him or her? Why now? Because definite answers may not be found, people often focus on particular things they did, or didn't do, or events that may have taken place just prior to diagnosis, or in the preceding months or years, that were in reality just coincidental

Staging
systems of classifying a patient's cancer by tumor size and how far it has spread in the body.

Cancer is in reality over 200 different diseases.

Malignancy
tumors that are characterized by the ability to invade surrounding tissue and spread to other parts of the body.

DNA (deoxyribonucleic acid)
the molecular building blocks of chromosomes. They contain and control genetic information in cells, including how they divide, grow, and function.

with regard to the cancer. If you or your loved one thinks that a particular event or situation caused the cancer, discuss these impressions with the doctor directly to gain a better understanding of the possible contributors to the cancer development and growth.

Misconceptions about cancer often arise when people generalize or misapply what very well may be true in limited cases. For example, although there is a virus associated with the development of cervical cancer, the cancer itself is not contagious. In fact, there are very few other cancers that originate in infectious processes. In a similar vein, although there is a genetic component to many cancers, there are almost always other factors involved that result in cancer actually developing; for this reason, one cannot simply say that cancer is inherited.

2. How is cancer treated?

The three major types of treatment traditionally have been **surgery**, **radiation therapy**, and **chemotherapy**. Surgery, which treats cancer by removing the cancerous tissue from the body (most often by cutting), is the oldest form of treatment. In the past, it was referred to as the "gold standard" of treatment because it was believed to be the treatment that most often led to a cure. Surgery, however, is not a treatment option for many cancers, such as leukemia and other blood cancers, or when the disease has spread throughout the body. And for other cancers such as prostate cancer, other treatments such as radiation therapy have been shown to be equally effective.

Radiation therapy, like surgery, targets specific areas in the body to treat. It employs high energy rays or sub-

Surgery
removal of a tumor, organ(s), or other objects from the body and/or repair of body parts using specific resection techniques.

Radiation therapy
used in both diagnosis and treatment, it is application of light, short radio waves, ultraviolet, or X-rays upon a specific area of the body for a period of time.

Chemotherapy
treatment of disease using chemical substances or drugs (also called "chemo").

atomic particles that damage the DNA of cancer cells and interfere with their growth, thereby shrinking the tumor, or eliminating it entirely. Chemotherapy also works by interfering with the growth and reproduction of cancer cells, but instead of radiation therapy, it uses toxic medications, the anticancer drugs. Chemotherapy differs from radiation therapy and surgery because it is most often a systemic therapy: instead of treating a part of the body, it treats cancer throughout the body. With all three major therapies—surgery, radiation therapy, and chemotherapy—a major issue has always been how to spare healthy tissue from the strong effects of the treatment; in other words, coping with the side effects. People equate chemotherapy, in particular, with nausea and hair loss, or radiation therapy with fatigue, but depending on the specific treatments—what medications are used or how the radiation therapy is administered—side effects can be controlled, reduced, or may not even occur at all.

In recent years promising new approaches to cancer treatment have been developed. One is immunotherapy or biological therapy, which utilizes parts of the body's own immune system to fight the disease. Gene therapy, on the other hand, attempts to fix cancer cells by replacing their missing or abnormal genes with normal ones, or blocking the genes that are important to the function or growth of the cancer cell. **Antiangiogenesis therapy** is another type of treatment that focuses on blocking the growth of new blood vessels to cancerous tumors, which they need to survive. What these experimental "targeted" therapies share is a much more precise approach to attacking the cancer, one that attempts to minimize the unintentional harm to healthy cells and tissues.

Antiangiogenesis therapy

experimental cancer treatment that focuses on blocking growth of new blood vessels to tumors.

There is continual refinement of the three traditional modes of treatment (surgery, radiation therapy, and chemotherapy). Together with the promise of the new approaches just outlined above, there is a greater sense of hope around the treatment and cure of cancer than there ever has been before. Cancer now is not the "dreaded disease" of the past that many people equated with death. Even though more cancer treatments exist and many types of cancer are being treated more effectively with greater change of cure, the fact remains that many cancers still come with poor **prognoses**. Even when treatments make it possible to think of some cancers as chronic conditions, these treatments can still challenge patients—as well as their families and friends—with their physical, emotional, and social demands. It is our belief that these challenges are met, in large part, through the education and support of the **caregivers** of the person with cancer.

There is a greater sense of hope around the treatment and cure of cancer than there ever has been before.

Prognosis
prediction of the course of a disease.

Caregiver
one who helps another person with a serious illness do what he or she ordinarily would be able to do, to meet his or her current and future needs.

3. What can I say to people who have cancer? What shouldn't I say?

You can say the same things you said to them before they had cancer. Don't be afraid to mention the disease, but attend closely to their responses. This means to listen not only to the words, but also the tone of voice and to observe body language. Some people want to talk about their cancer, while others don't. And how they respond today can change the next time you see them, so it's not a bad idea to check in with them occasionally by asking again if they'd like to talk. If they prefer not to discuss their cancer, at least they know you care and are willing to listen when they're ready. Besides, it's not always necessary to talk about the cancer, and surely there are many other things that they would enjoy having a conversation about.

If and when a person with cancer does decide to talk, it may be better simply to listen well to what he or she has to say rather than to say things you think will make the person feel better. If you want to say something encouraging, remind the person of his or her personal strengths or how well he or she had survived hard times in the past. Focus on really listening to what the person with cancer says. Rephrase what he or she has told you and say it back to him or her. This type of communication may seem unnatural to you at first, but it can be an effective way to demonstrate that you are listening to what the person is saying.

It may be better simply to listen.

Try not to offer advice unless it is asked for. Keep in mind that talking about other people you know who have had the same diagnosis or a comparable illness may come across as second-guessing the specific decisions a person with cancer has made or as a criticism of how he or she has handled the experience in general. Do not stop calling or visiting, unless he or she specifically tells you to stop communicating. And, do not tell others about the diagnosis or the information shared with you unless you have the patient's permission. Trust is particularly important at this time.

Mark's comment:

Basically, when a friend or relative tells you they have cancer, there's not much you can or even should say—you just have to try to listen to them. When a male friend of mine, Frank, explained to me about his lymphoma, I didn't really say much except that I thought he should go get a second opinion—it didn't seem as though his doctor was telling him what he needed to know. After asking him first, I then I made an effort to go out and find some good doctors who came highly recommended. Frank is not knowledgeable about computers or the Internet, so doing it for him saved him some trouble. I don't ask him about his cancer—I let him talk about it when he wants to.

There are a lot of things you shouldn't say. If hearing your friend has cancer makes you uncomfortable, you might react by being overly sympathetic and alarmed, or else joke the discomfort away, and neither response is very helpful. It's best to be matter-of-fact about the subject and supportive, urging the person to talk if he or she wants to. Humor does have its place—there are times that being blunt, in a humorous way, can help your friend to cope better. For example, a female friend, Janet, who has a brain tumor, was waffling about going through with her surgery because, she said, "I don't want to be bald." I told her, "Bald is temporary, dead is permanent." And she laughed. But then she admitted what I already had figured out, which was that she was scared of dying during surgery, and I let her talk about that. Although talking didn't change her mind any about the surgery—she still hasn't had it, and every day she procrastinates risks her life—but at least she can talk about her real fears now and isn't quite so scared of the prospect.

4. How do I offer to help a person with cancer?

Mark's comment:

When I was caring for my mother, and now that I have two friends with cancer, I have made a habit of offering whatever seemed to make sense in the situation. I've bought groceries for them, given them rides to different places they might need to go—things like that. I did a lot of shopping for my mother, but I tried not to take over her life too much because she hated being dependent on other people. And she was a proper Yankee lady, so there were certain things she didn't want her son doing for her anyway—like her laundry, or bathing her. I just did the things I could to help out around the house without making her feel like she wasn't independent anymore.

If you would like to do something to help a person with cancer, it's often easier to suggest specific and concrete ways of providing help, rather than making an open-ended offer of "Just let me know if you need anything." Try asking if you can bring over a meal that week, do laundry, or take him or her to an appointment. You can also do errands for the immediate family, such as grocery shopping or taking in the car for an oil change—anything to free them up to devote more time to attend to the needs of the person with cancer.

Suggest specific and concrete ways of providing help.

When offering to help, it's important to be flexible. The kind of help that is offered or expected is often related to how the giver and receiver of help view their relationship with one another. For example, most people would not be comfortable with a casual acquaintance offering to take their kids for the summer. If your offer of help is turned down, however, it may be for reasons that have nothing to do with you or the relationship. So don't be offended. Offer to do something else you believe the person may be more comfortable with, and, of course, make sure that it's something that you yourself are comfortable doing.

5. What does it mean to be a "caregiver"?

A caregiver is someone who helps another person to do things that ordinarily he would be able to do by himself. There are professional caregivers such as nurses and nursing attendants who provide this care as a formal service for pay. Then there are the millions of informal caregivers, including family members and friends, who provide this assistance without expecting to be paid a fee. Done out of love, friendship, or duty, the rewards for these informal caregivers are not monetary, even though the value of the care was an estimated 257 billion dollars a year in 2002.

Stated in such a way, it would seem that a "caregiver" provides practical assistance only with the activities of daily living. In reality, the role is much broader. A caregiver often has the responsibility of coordinating the person's medical needs and appointments. This coordination may include finding the right doctors to diagnose and treat the disease, helping the patient get to the best places to provide medical treatment, and, if needed, then accessing and utilizing rehabilitative therapies after treatment. And just as importantly, the caregiver monitors the person's emotional well-being, providing direct support or helping him or her to get **counseling** as needed.

Counseling
mental health therapy with a professionally trained therapist.

Caregivers, therefore, fulfill a wide range of functions by identifying and helping to meet the needs of the person with cancer. If you see yourself as a caregiver, your roles can vary widely and may include being a partner, acting as a nurse, a housekeeper, a cook, a psychologist, a chauffeur, a secretary, or performing another role. Sometimes, you may not know which role to play at any given time. The challenge of being a caregiver is taking on tasks that you never expected and may have had no preparation for. Being asked to do something that you do not feel competent to handle can be frightening and frustrating. Being asked to

The challenge of being a caregiver is taking on tasks that you never expected.

do ten new things for a loved one, and not knowing when or if you'll ever be relieved of the responsibility for doing them, can be a source of significant stress and tension. However, preparing yourself—reading this book, investigating other resources, and discussing these duties with medical care professionals—can reduce anxiety associated with caregiver responsibilities. The first step is knowing that there is information, emotional support, and other services available to help you if you feel overwhelmed.

6. Why did I become the caregiver?

Mark's comment:

I became the primary caregiver for my mother because I was the only relative who lived nearby, and I was also the one who was emotionally closest to her. After I reached adulthood, I had become as much a friend to her as a son. I was also fortunate enough to be self-employed, which allowed me a great deal of flexibility in my time. But even if that hadn't been the case, as far as I was concerned, it was my responsibility as her son to take care of her when she was sick. That was a good enough reason for me.

There is an expectation in our society that a person with a life-threatening illness will have someone to assume the role of **primary caregiver**. Most often this is a spouse (or "significant other") or an adult child for an older patient. When family, either by blood or marriage, is unavailable, we often look to close friends to provide essential support.

Although the caregiver role would seem to fall on the person who has the closest relationship with the

Primary caregiver
one who personally provides, or organizes others to provide, the essential logistical and emotional support for a person with cancer.

patient, a number of other factors influence the decision as to who will take on the primary caregiving responsibility. Proximity, or simply living close by, may be one reason why it was decided that you as opposed to your sister, who lives farther away, would be your mother's caregiver. Of course, the patient may have asked you to help simply because he or she trusts you and believes you'll do a good job. Or, you may have volunteered for this role as primary caregiver because it is a role you feel comfortable with.

Many people, despite the shock and dismay of having a loved one diagnosed with cancer, find solace and deep personal satisfaction in being a primary caregiver. It is a role that allows them to demonstrate, through the care they provide, their love and esteem for the patient. Also, it feels good to be helpful and feel needed by a loved one.

For others, their reaction to caregiving might be more ambivalent. Because of a history of strained family relationships, they may wonder "why me?" They may feel pressure not only from family members, but also from co-workers, acquaintances, and members of the health-care team as well, to provide care, regardless of their desire or perceived ability to do so. If you became the primary caregiver because of other people's expectations, it is important that you are aware of these expectations and your own feelings about the matter. Mixed feelings at the beginning about your role can lead to a greater sense of frustration later on, so it is important to acknowledge your limits as early as possible before they become problematic, so that you and the patient can make alternative care arrangements, if possible.

PART TWO

Managing Medical Treatment and Care

We have met so many people involved in my wife's care. Who are all these people, and what do they do?

Who is the best doctor to treat this cancer? How do I find that doctor?

When should we seek a second opinion?

More ...

7. We have met so many people involved in my wife's care. Who are all these people, and what do they do?

The health care team is composed of different professionals who are specially trained to deal with the medical and emotional issues you are confronting. Become familiar with these people and the ways they can help you. Below is a list of the standard team members and what they can do for you:

Oncologist

physician expert in the treatment of cancer; includes overseeing administration of chemotherapy and other regimens.

Radiation oncologist

physician expert in radiation therapy.

Registered nurse (RN)

Provides patient care; usually has completed a four-year college degree and hospital training.

Nurse Practitioner (NP)

advanced practice clinician with a master's degree who can prescribe medications and write medical orders.

Clinical nurse specialist (CNS)

nurse with a master's degree who can provide patient care and education in a medical specialty.

- Physicians and surgeons (MDs). May include a medical **oncologist** (expert in chemotherapy, among other cancer treatments), a surgeon, and/or a **radiation oncologist** (expert in radiation therapy). There are many additional doctors and specialists who may be involved in determining the diagnosis of cancer and/or its treatment. If you are unfamiliar with the different terms used to describe these specialists, feel free to ask these professionals for clarification.

- Nurses. **Registered nurses** (RNs) typically have a four-year college degree and hospital training. They are an integral part of patient care and will be extremely helpful to you. Nurses provide patient care on the inpatient floors and outpatient centers, and they can be very specialized in the type of care they provide. A **nurse practitioner** (NP) is an advanced practice clinician with a master's degree who, under supervision of a doctor, can prescribe medications and write medical orders in most states, provide direct medical care, and serve as a good resource for important information. A **clinical nurse specialist** (CNS) is a nurse with a master's degree who can provide patient care, but also specializes in the role of an educator in a medical specialty. Depending on your state and hospital policies, other people may be involved in different types of hands-on patient care, including **licensed practical nurses** (LPN), nursing assistants, and patient certified technicians (PCT).

- **Physician Assistants** (PA). PAs are medical professionals that can diagnose, treat, and write prescriptions and medical orders, all under the supervision of a physician. Many clinics and hospitals employ both PAs and NPs to assist the physicians treating cancer.

- **Social Workers**. In most states, certified or licensed social workers (CSW, LCSW, LSW) usually have at least a master's degree (MSW, MSSW). They are available to assist you in coping with the diagnosis, the stress of adjustment to treatment and hospitalization, and can provide counseling to patients and their families. They also may help identify community resources and may coordinate patient discharge from the hospital.

- **Case Managers** (or discharge planners). Some hospitals have nurse case managers who are responsible for coordinating discharge from the hospital, whereas at other hospitals social workers perform this role. Find out who performs this role at your hospital so that you can contact that person to discuss home care, equipment, placement (e.g., **nursing home**), or other discharge needs when your loved one goes home.

- **Interns/residents/fellows**. If your loved one is being treated at a teaching hospital, he or she may have a variety of "doctors-in-training." These team members often can be helpful and supportive of you. Remember, however, that the **attending physician** is the person who is in charge of a hospital patient's care, and that if you have questions or

Licensed practical nurse (LPN)

has completed a two-year degree in nursing; often involved with hands-on patient care.

Physician Assistant (PA)

medical professional who can diagnose, treat and write prescriptions under a physician's guidance.

Social Workers

certified or licensed social workers (CSW, LCSW, LSW) usually have a master's degree (MSW, MSSW) or doctorate (DSW, PhD), and counsel the patient and family coping with the stress of diagnosis and treatment. These professionals also can identify community mental health resources and many coordinate patient discharge.

Case Manager

also called a discharge planner. Nurse or social worker who coordinates the patient's discharge from a hospital.

Nursing home

facility that provides long-term custodial care for patients who can no longer live at home.

Intern

physician-in-training working in a teaching hospital.

Attending physician

physician in charge of a hospital patient's care.

Dietitian

a professional who plans tailored diets to meet the nutritional requirements of people with special health care needs.

think that you have been given inconsistent information, you can ask to speak directly to the attending physician in charge of your loved one's care.

- Clinical **Dietitians/Nutritionists**. They are available to provide education on the role of diet in a patient's recovery from cancer. They are often part of the inpatient team and sometimes are available in outpatient clinics as well. You may want to contact one of these professionals to answer any questions you may have on what foods to eat, preparation of food, and any foods your loved one should avoid during or after treatments.

Hospitals also employ many other experts who may be involved in your spouse's care, such as patient advocates/representatives, physical therapists, respiratory therapists, occupational therapists, psychologists, psychiatrists, other physician specialists, hospital chaplains, technicians, and patient escorts. It is often helpful for you and your loved one to get to know these people. By making a personal connection, you may feel more comfortable and supported by those around you.

8. Who is the best doctor to treat this cancer? How do I find that doctor?

People use different criteria when choosing a physician. Many factors will influence people's decisions, including the physician's experience treating cancer and his or her technical skills, the hospital's location, insurance coverage, and personal factors, such as the physician's ability to gain trust and confidence (or "bedside manner"). Interview physicians; assess their experience

Managing Medical Treatment and Care

and other criteria that you and your loved one consider important. If you have just received the diagnosis of cancer, you and the patient may consider seeking a second opinion from a cancer specialist in your area, ideally from a physician who routinely treats cancer.

Finding the right doctor is sometimes stressful. If you do not already have a doctor to treat your cancer, you may want to ask your primary care physician for a referral. National organizations can also help you find an appropriate physician. We have provided a list of Internet resources that may be helpful in your doctor search (see the Appendix for a list of resources). Additionally, if you are comfortable, ask family or friends for the names of oncologists they know and liked. We provide several resources you may use to locate cancer specialists (see the Appendix). You may also contact your insurance company for a referral suggestion.

Questions to ask a doctor:

1. **Years of experience treating cancer** *(How long have you been treating patients with cancer?)*

2. **Specialization** *(Are you experienced in treating the type of cancer my loved one has? If so, how many cases do you treat a year? Are you involved in researching new treatments for this type of cancer?)*

3. **Communication** *(If I have questions, how should I let you know?)*

4. **Insurance plan coverage** *(Do you participate with my insurance policy? If not, then what are alternative payment options?)*

5. **Proposed treatment plans** *(What is (are) the goal(s) of treatment? What are the various treatment options?)*

9. When should we seek a second opinion?

Mark's comment:

When my mother was diagnosed with colon cancer twenty years ago, we knew that there was a really good clinic (hospital) to go to for treatment in our area, so we went there. But my mother interviewed a number of doctors at the clinic until she found one she was comfortable with—the decision had nothing to do with me. As a physician's widow, she was fairly well equipped to do her own questioning, so she did it and I didn't try to interfere. Back then there weren't that many cancer specialists, and she questioned the clinic's doctors very thoroughly. With my friends Frank and Janet, who were diagnosed more recently, we did some Internet research and asked people familiar with cancer treatment to recommend someone. There are a lot of big-name cancer treatment centers in the Boston area, so we started with those. Frank ended up switching from his first doctor to someone at a renowned cancer specialty hospital and was much happier with the treatment he got. As for Janet, it turned out that the surgical oncologist that Janet's doctor had referred her to was the same man who came most highly recommended by a brain surgeon my wife knew, so that worked out pretty well.

Some people are comfortable with the treatment options presented by the first physician they consult. However, patients get second opinions from other doctors for many reasons, and seeking another opinion should be viewed positively by the original doctor. You may seek another opinion due to insurance company requirements, because your loved one is diagnosed with a rare or advanced cancer, or simply because you feel most comfortable exploring more options.

You may wish to seek a second opinion from a specialist at a large cancer research center. Some people decide to have their treatment at the cancer specialty hospital, but others get second opinions and then decide to undergo treatment locally, depending on the recommendations and treatment options. Many oncologists believe that a second opinion should be standard for every new cancer diagnosis.

Seeking a second opinion can be helpful when deciding between or among different treatment options. Be sure to take all medical records with you, including copies of X-ray films, pathology/diagnostic reports and/or other information about the cancer (or suspected) diagnosis, or the person's medical history. If the information or recommendation provided by the physicians is confusing, discuss your concerns and questions with the involved physicians openly so that they can address your questions up-front. If necessary, you may wish to seek multiple opinions; be careful, however, that medical treatment is not delayed too long since the timing of medical intervention is sometimes an important factor in determining its appropriateness for use.

10. Between appointments, my wife and I think of many important questions to ask the doctor, but when we finally get into the exam room, I get intimidated

and distracted. How can I be more relaxed and better express myself to the medical team?

One of the many ways caregivers support patients is by attending appointments with them. The relationship you have with the medical team is a crucial aspect of patient care and can be most helpful when dealing with important treatment decisions. If you are feeling vulnerable, there are several things you can do to make yourself more comfortable:

- Before you go to a doctor's appointment, the two of you should discuss your questions and concerns in advance. By preparing a list of questions before you step into the office, you will be less likely to forget any important topics you wish to discuss.
- Record by date any physical observations about your loved one since your last visit, such as the possible side effects of treatment or medications, including pain, fatigue, nausea, sleeplessness, and/or any other body changes. Also, encourage open discussion with your wife's doctor about her coping, particularly if she is feeling sad, depressed, or anxious.
- Encourage your loved one to be *honest* with the team about her symptoms and about how she is feeling. We have known some patients to want to "hide" side effects of their treatment for many reasons. For example, they may think that the doctor will put them on a lower dose of treatment, which will make it less likely to cure the cancer, or they fear that their cancer is growing if they feel bad. Still other people are concerned about appearing "weak" to the doctor.

Encourage your loved one to be honest with the team.

- Document the doctor's answers and instructions, or use a tape recorder so that you will remember important points after you leave the exam room. Be sure to ask your doctor's permission first before using recording devices.

- Ask for clarification if you do not understand what the doctor is saying. Oncology physicians are experts in treating cancer, but sometimes they communicate differently than other people do. If you do not understand, do not feel embarrassed to ask, ask, and ask again. Nurses are specially trained to educate you about medical issues and can address many concerns. Asking the clinical nurse to clarify information in plain terms can be extremely helpful.

- If necessary, ask someone with whom you and the patient are comfortable to come with you so that you have another person listening to what the doctor says. This person can serve as support and as your advocate, particularly if you have concerns about expressing yourself or feel overwhelmed by the information.

- Identify what you think and how you feel about the doctor. Is he or she intimidating, or likable? Does the doctor use complex terms that you don't understand? Are you afraid of what he or she will find or say about the cancer? Answers to such questions can point you in the right direction for overcoming any negative feelings you may have. Discuss concerns you have directly with the physician. In doing this, many problems can be solved, which can help you feel more comfortable. If your feelings are interfering with your ability to get appropriate medical care for your loved one, you and your wife may consider finding another physician more suited to the both of you.

11. My wife and I don't speak English well. What can we do to make sure this doesn't become a problem?

Linguistic, ethnic, and cultural differences may exist between you and the medical team; these differences may make communication difficult and add to any initial uncertainty you may feel. If you have questions or concerns about these issues, talk to your hospital social worker, patient representative or advocate, or another health care professional with whom you feel comfortable.

If your primary language is not English and your loved one is being treated in the United States, your anxiety may be even higher because of difficulty in communication. Try to bring a family or friend who can interpret for you. Keep in mind that you and your wife want to feel as comfortable as possible discussing personal information required in some doctors' visits, so be sure that the person translating is someone you trust and through whom you can communicate openly. Additionally, many hospitals have staff or volunteer translators available. If they do not, investigate buying an electronic translator or an electronic dictionary, particularly for use in emergency situations. Phone translation services are also available from some companies, such as LanguageLine Services (see the Appendix for contact information). In fact, some consent forms are available in other languages. If you do not understand what the doctors are saying, or need further clarification, urge your loved one not to consent to medical treatment until she fully understands.

12. Playing the "hurry up and wait" game—why does it take so long to do a workup or to see the doctor?

One of the most common complaints we hear from patients and their caregivers is about waiting. Waiting for test results, waiting to see the doctor, waiting for procedures, and more waiting. Waiting to see doctors is so common that we as patients come to expect it. However, after a cancer diagnosis, when you may have many appointments, or go regularly to the hospital, this waiting can become particularly annoying. Coupled with the already higher stress levels, waiting can be extremely frustrating.

There are many reasons for the long waits. Sometimes tests or preparation is required before some procedures, such as blood work before receiving chemotherapy. Other times, paperwork needs to be processed, including the doctor's specific medical orders, or tests (including X-rays and other lab work) need to be fully reviewed before a patient sees the doctor. There is a lot of "behind-the-scenes" work being done on your loved one's behalf, so keep this in mind when you are waiting to see the doctor or to receive a medical test and/or treatment. Furthermore, some hospitals and physicians are very busy and see as many patients as possible in a given day. This is good because more people can be examined and treated by the doctor, but it also can mean longer waits if things get backed up or emergencies occur.

Finding productive ways to pass the time can be good as these activities lower stress levels. Bring a good book, magazine(s), CDs/tapes, a simple game (playing cards) or crafts (such as knitting or crocheting), along with snacks and water for both you and the patient. You also may consider bringing a sweater/jacket (for cold offices) and/or a small pillow (for hard seats or to support the lower back). We have known caregivers to bring work from their offices to feel productive or review personal research they have done about cancer treatments or coping with cancer.

Despite the distractions, keep in mind that you are there to provide reassurance and support to your loved one. You may want to use the waiting time to talk to one another about what questions to ask the doctor, or about how each other is feeling, both physically (for the patient) and emotionally (for both of you).

If you are comfortable, start a conversation with another patient and/or caregiver. Some family members have met fellow caregivers for other patients in the waiting areas. Speaking with others can be helpful in gathering useful information. It also helps you realize that others are facing similar experiences.

If you are waiting a long time and/or your loved one is feeling unwell, let the nurse or receptionist know, especially if the patient is experiencing increased pain, fever, nausea, or sudden onset of other physical symptoms.

13. Where can I find reliable information about cancer?

There are a number of sources for reliable information as noted below:

a. Your doctor(s), including your primary care physician, medical oncologist, surgeon, and other physician specialists should be your primary source of information.

b. Nurses and other medical staff (see Question 7)

c. Books based on sound medical advice (see the Appendix under "Recommended Books")

d. Pamphlets/brochures often are available from your doctor/nurse, but you also can order them directly (see the Appendix).

e. The Internet is a valuable resource for information. However, be very careful to gather information from reliable Web sites, including the National Cancer Institute, American Cancer Society, or Cancer Care (see Questions 14 and the Appendix).

f. Family, friends, and others closest to you may have useful tips, resources, and other information for you to investigate. However, take such advice from non-professionals with a "grain of salt," so to speak. It is best to investigate for yourself.

g. TV/radio/magazines/newspaper: The media reports on many "medical breakthroughs" in cancer research and treatment. Some of this information can be informative. Consider keeping a file of newspaper or magazine articles, or notes about information you hear from other media sources. Then discuss them with your doctor. Unfortunately, sometimes the research reported is too preliminary to be helpful or relates to medical situations different than what your loved one is experiencing.

14. Are chat rooms and Internet postings good places to look for information?

We recommend many Internet sites, not only for information about the medical aspects of cancer, but also for information about coping with cancer, including the family, emotional, financial, and work-related issues that often accompany the diagnosis. Furthermore, chat rooms and other Web site postings can provide useful tips on locating information, finding doctors who treat specific types of cancer, and discussing many other concerns you may have.

Many patients and caregivers have found the Internet a very valuable resource, empowering them with information that may be particularly helpful in the beginning of the diagnosis and when making treatment decisions. On the other hand, too much information can be overwhelming, particularly when the information is riddled with unfamiliar medical terms. Even recommended and reliable Web sites such as the National Cancer Institute (NCI; *www.cancer.gov*) can be confusing given the complex and technical nature of the information provided.

Importantly, the Internet has increasingly become a source of emotional support for patients and caregivers. For example, the American Cancer Society (*www.cancer.org*) offers a variety of "Message Boards" focused on many topics that may be helpful. Cancer Care, Inc. offers online **support groups**, including one called "Caregiver Empowerment Support Group," which provides emotional support for family members of people with cancer. These resources also offer other online support services to patients.

Support group
a gathering that is focused on sharing experiences, providing emotional support, and relieving the sense of isolation. May be led by social workers or trained cancer survivor volunteers.

Be aware that there are many Web sites providing false information and unsubstantiated claims, or selling unproven remedies for profit. There are many unconventional theories about cancer, its treatment, and how to best cope with this disease, and not all of these theories are helpful. In fact, some of the methods proposed are potentially harmful. Keep in mind that you need to read everything with a critical mind, and do not necessarily believe personal testimonials, single reports of "new cures," or any other sources of information that are not backed by a doctor you trust. Be particularly wary of purchasing anything. If you hear about something particularly interesting, do more research on the topic using the recommended resources suggested in the Appendix, and discuss all information with your doctor(s).

You need to read everything with a critical mind.

15. It seems the more we find out, the more questions we have. Can too much information be a problem?

Some family members cope well by learning everything possible about the cancer and its treatment. However, there is a bewildering amount of information out there—on the Internet, TV, radio, and newspapers—and being bombarded with all of these sources can contribute to feeling overwhelmed. Additionally, diagnosing and treating cancer are complicated processes, often necessitating specialists to understand all this information. As a nonmedical professional, you cannot be expected to read and understand all of these details in the short time you have to make a decision.

Start by reading information given to you by the physician. Review this information and then discuss it with the doctor. If you have more questions or wish to do more research, investigate legitimate resources (see the Appendix). Write down questions as they come to you, and then organize them according to subject. This not only will help you organize questions for the doctor but may make you feel less overwhelmed by making your questions seem more manageable. Keep in mind that not all questions can be answered. Medicine simply cannot answer all questions about treatment effectiveness or side effects, since so many individual differences occur. If no answer is available and you have discussed it with the physician, try to accept this and move forward. A cancer diagnosis is a venture into the unknown, for both the person with cancer and family.

Keep in mind that not all questions can be answered.

16. What are clinical trials? How do we locate appropriate trials?

Advances in treating cancer often start in a scientific laboratory where potential therapies are first developed and tested. When one of these potential therapies shows promise in treating cancer, it is tested in many ways, including using animals to determine its possible effectiveness and safety. If the potential therapy passes these tests, then it goes through a series of strict government reviews for human safety. After it is reviewed by many physicians and scientists, and receives government approval, it then may be offered to human volunteers for further testing. These volunteers are sometimes referred to as "research participants," or by the outdated term, "research subjects."

Experimental protocol

research of a new drug or therapy using very specific materials and steps.

Research participants who meet very specific medical criteria (such as cancer diagnosis, stage of disease, and many other factors) may be eligible to participate in an **experimental protocol**. One type of experimental protocol is a clinical trial, which tests cancer treatments on people. Clinical trials may test brand-new treatments, or may involve treatments that already are in use to treat other diseases or cancer types, but physicians want to see if the therapy may be effective with different types of cancer. Or, doctors may want to test a new combination of treatments to improve effectiveness when combined. Clinical trials are the backbone of advances in treating cancer and other diseases. If your family member decides to participate in one, he or she will not only get state-of-the-art treatment, but also will be playing a meaningful role in advancing cancer treatments, with the potential to save other people's lives.

Clinical trials are primarily conducted at large research hospitals and are often supported by pharmaceutical companies and government research funds. However, trials can sometimes be offered at private physicians' offices and other non-specialty hospitals. Participants are often needed to enroll in clinical trials; in fact, some trials have a hard time getting enough people to enroll primarily because patients don't know they exist. If you are interested in investigating clinical trials, a good first step is your local oncologist or primary care physician—whoever is discussing treatment options with you. However, physicians may not be aware of all the hundreds of clinical trials open at any given time, so you may want to do some research on your own and then discuss your findings with the doctor. Three excellent resources are the American Cancer Society (ACS), the National Cancer Institute (NCI), and the Cancer Information Service (CIS). ACS and NCI both have searchable databases online that provide descriptions of the research, general eligibility criteria, and contact information. CIS allows you to call by telephone to obtain similar information (see the Appendix for contact information).

17. Is it better to be in a clinical trial rather than standard treatment?

This is a hard question to answer, since clinical trials entail different potential benefits and risks depending on the individual, the cancer diagnosis and stage, and the treatment proposed. People often believe that they will get more scientifically advanced treatment if they enroll in a clinical trial. Some people with advanced disease who want treatment may only have the option of enrolling in a clinical trial if standard treatments are not available.

Clinical trials usually involve more frequent check-ups and detailed interviews regarding symptoms than traditional treatment follow-up to make sure that the treatment is working properly and is without significant side effects. And, since clinical trials are often performed at major cancer centers, patients may believe they are getting the state-of-the-art treatment for their cancer, which is often the case.

Keep in mind, however, that the treatment involved in clinical trials may have side effects, as any cancer treatment does, but sometimes the effects of these treatments involved in clinical trials are not as well known as standard cancer therapy. Therefore, make sure your loved one enters a clinical trial with "eyes open," understanding all the pros and cons of the proposed study including possible harm and side effects, and potential benefits. This research may benefit other patients being

Make sure your loved one enters a clinical trial with "eyes open."

treated in the future by allowing doctors to test new and potentially better treatments.

18. Will my insurance pay for treatment in a clinical trial?

It is a good idea to contact the insurance company directly to determine whether the patient's insurance policy will cover therapy involved in clinical trials. Some insurance companies will pay for all treatment expenses, including any added costs associated with clinical trials (if there are any). At the other extreme, insurance companies may decline to pay for any treatment considered "experimental" or therapy that is part of a clinical trial. Other policies are somewhere in between; some states have enacted legislation mandating that private insurance companies pay for treatment involved in clinical trials (see the American Cancer Society [ACS] Web site for details). However, a patient may be responsible for the costs above and beyond what would have accrued with standard treatment. **Medicare**, for example, may have coverage restrictions for treatments that are part of clinical trials (see Question 77). Understand that the patient may be responsible for the balance. If you do run into financial roadblocks with entering a clinical trial, appeal to the insurance company and/or seek assistance from your doctor or social worker, as sometimes there is additional funding for some **protocols** to assist people with the added expenses.

Medicare
federally run health insurance program for those aged 65 or more, on Social Security Disability, legally blind, or on renal dialysis.

Protocol
description of a clinical trial; also used more generally to refer to a plan of medical treatment.

19. How do I know whether we are making the best treatment decisions?

After the initial diagnosis, people with cancer and their families have to make medical decisions and sometimes are uncertain about what the "right" decisions may be. As the patient and family are making important decisions, stress levels are higher. A huge amount of information about cancer must be absorbed. People differ in how much they want to know about the cancer, such as stage of disease, progression, and so on. If you or the patient is the type of person who would rather not know the details, designate one or two family members to attend appointments with you to gather necessary information. These individuals can serve as "point persons" through whom the medical team can communicate openly.

Always discuss external information sources directly with the doctor, who is a partner in the patient's care. Topics of discussion with the doctor may include personal research from books or the Internet. *Do not* rely solely on Internet chat rooms, personal testimonials, or the thousands of cancer resources that exist, because many of them are unreliable (see the Appendix containing reliable, useful resources at the end of this book). Even on reliable Web sites, statistics and medical information can be confusing and shocking. Filter all information through your doctor to get the real story, clarify concerns, and get the answers to all questions regarding treatment.

The patient and family may be presented with several options regarding treatment, and the physician will leave the final decision up to the patient. Some patients like being able to make this decision because they feel that they are actively involved in their own care. Others, however, are confused and anxious about making such important medical decisions, and this may be true for their partners and caregivers as well. It is important that you and the patient get clarification on the pros and cons of different treatment options from the medical team, including the factors that affect the quality of life of the patient. For example, does one chemotherapy regimen have more side effects than the other, even though both may be equally effective in treating the cancer?

Get clarification on the pros and cons of different treatment options from the medical team.

Clarifying the issues, having support, and sharing the burden of decision-making between the patient and yourself can take pressure off both of you. However, remember that the patient should have the final say, as it is he or she who must live with whatever decisions are made. You may never know the one "right" decision to make, as is common with many decisions in life. Don't put too much pressure on yourselves. Make an informed decision with the assistance of the medical team and then move forward.

20. My husband says that he would rather die than live with the surgery the doctors suggest. Can't he just let his disease take its natural course without subjecting himself to this treatment?

Being diagnosed with cancer is a tremendous burden on anyone, and the ability to cope with feelings may be more difficult if someone is told that a permanent (or even temporary) physical change may be necessary. For example, most people do not want to live with an **ostomy** (which entails wearing a "bag" to collect bowel movements or urine), or having their breast removed (**mastectomy**), or a **prostatectomy** (removal of the prostate, which can alter men's physical/sexual responses), or

Ostomy
surgery to create an opening from the skin to the urinary or gastrointestinal canal, or the trachea.

Mastectomy
surgical removal of the breast.

Prostatectomy
surgical removal of part or all of the prostate.

other surgeries that change the look and/or function of their bodies. Some people may consider declining surgery or other treatments, such as chemotherapy or radiation therapy.

If your spouse is having a similar reaction to a proposed treatment, help him take a step back and review his decision-making process so that he can be sure that he is making the best decisions. Patients need to weigh their own values when making any treatment decision, including whether or not to have treatment at all. Some people who initially decline a procedure later change their minds, after the initial shock subsides. Sometimes taking the time to talk more to the physician, talking to other people who have had the same procedure or treatment, and/or seeking a second opinion can help ease this decision-making process. Use this added information to help your loved one make the right medical decisions for him. Encourage him to research his choice and to take control over his decisions.

When discussing the pros and cons of an operation with a surgeon, ask about the location and reason for surgery or treatment, and confirm the need for the particular medical intervention that has been proposed as opposed to other options. If it is indeed recommended, and you and your partner are still unsure of whether or not to proceed, make sure that you are aware of the consequences.

It is important that you understand that "letting nature take its course" does not necessarily mean slipping gradually into a gentle death. For example, not having a surgery such as a **colostomy** can result in medical complications, including possible obstruction of the colon and tumor invasion of other organs, potentially resulting in lower quality of life including pain and frequent hospitalizations. Foregoing surgery or treatment can hasten a patient's death.

Sometimes patients and family members disagree about whether the patient should undergo the treatments/surgery the doctors offer or suggest. Occasionally, family members are adamant that the patient undergo the procedure despite the patient's reservations or explicit refusal. If this describes your situation, first, talk to your spouse about why he has made this decision. Be sure to listen—not argue—with the reasons. Then, after your spouse has finished, explain your point of view as calmly as possible, understanding that the final decision is his to make, but that the decision does affect the rest of the family. If tensions are high, then you and he may want to talk to a trusted friend or a more impartial person, such as a nurse, counselor, minister, or social worker, to help focus the conversations and keep the lines of communication open.

Furthermore, be aware what your reasons are for wanting your husband to have the suggested treatment. As social workers, we have seen family members sometimes fear the loss of their loved one so much that they are willing to do anything to keep him or her alive. Sometimes the proposed treatments can be invasive and lead to side effects that may not be worth the suffering to the patient. You need to consider your feelings because you, too, are affected by your husband's

Colostomy

surgery to establish an artificial connection between the lumen of the colon and the skin.

Managing Medical Treatment and Care

diagnosis, but be sure that your opinions are based on a fair assessment of his wishes as well.

21. My adult daughter always seems to be complaining of being in pain or fatigue and generally not feeling well. I don't think that she is trying hard enough. Are her "unseen" symptoms real? If so, what can I do to help her?

Yes, most likely her symptoms are real. Listening to your daughter's complaints may be making you feel frustrated and helpless, particularly if this has been going on for a while and progress has been slow. Sometimes, in order to reduce their own feelings of not being able to help, family and friends try to minimize the situation. However, no one can say how much pain, fatigue, or distress your daughter feels, except your daughter herself. It is very important that you believe what your daughter is saying, particularly about her pain, because when people in pain think that no one believes them, this increases their distress. As a result, they may stop telling others exactly what is happening with their pain, which then makes the pain more difficult to control.

Most pain can be relieved to the degree that allows patients to live a reasonable life, though it may require patience and persistence to find the right regimen. Sometimes pain is directly connected with a cancer tumor, which when treated through surgery, radiation therapy, and/or chemotherapy, reduces the source of the pain itself. Medication, including analgesics like acetaminophen and ibuprofen, as well as more powerful opioid drugs like morphine and oxycodone, can be used on a regular basis to prevent pain from beginning, in addition to keeping it under control. And there is a host of other measures—from warm baths and hot water bottles to relaxation exercises and training in guided imagery—that will not only help to reduce your daughter's feelings of pain, but will also help to increase her sense of control with regard to it. Talking about her pain in detail and on a regular basis should not be thought of as "dwelling on it," but as a necessary way of getting accurate information to the medical team members so that they can effectively and promptly treat it.

Psychological distress is common among people in pain. And, it is also possible that there are other psychological issues, such as depression and anxiety, which are contributing to your daughter's expressions of pain and fatigue. To support the person with cancer, it is better to address psychological factors separately from her physical complaints, at least in the beginning. We've outlined elsewhere in this book how to evaluate emotional distress in your loved one, ways to gauge the seriousness of the distress and options for treatment (see Questions 31–33). The person with cancer first needs to know that she has a care partner she can trust, someone who hears her specific complaints and is working with her to find solutions.

If your daughter's pain continues, help her communicate this to her doctor and persist in finding methods of relief. Since our expertise as social workers does not focus on the management of physical symptoms and possible treatment side effects, we suggest that you or your daughter contact the doctor's office immediately if new or unresolved symptoms occur. Furthermore, a very useful resource on managing physical issues at home is published by the American Cancer Society and is available on their Web site ("Caring for the Patient with Cancer at Home"; see the Appendix for details).

22. I sometimes feel that I am doing too much for my father. The doctors and the physical therapist say that he needs to do more for himself, including walking, preparing meals, and other things. How can I allow my father to do these things without feeling that I am neglecting him?

A cancer diagnosis and treatments change a person's body, sometimes making it difficult to resume past activities. Sometimes these changes are permanent, but sometimes physical changes such as fatigue or weakness can be improved. Ask your father's doctor and physical therapist what they mean, exactly, when they say they want him "to do more for himself." Ask them to help establish reasonable and specific goals for your father, in order to increase his activity slowly.

Find out what he believes his limitations are.

The most important part of this process is how your father feels about his own abilities. Sometimes patients worry about physical symptoms, or fear that they will hurt themselves. Find out what he believes his limitations are and why he has them. If his concerns are medical in nature, try to have the medical team address them with him directly. Then you can work out a plan with your father on how to get him to do the activities the medical team recommends. Be flexible. It may take time, or trial periods of alternative or intermediate activities, before your father reaches the goals you've agreed upon. But by making your father a partner in the process, you help enhance his self-esteem and relieve yourself of feeling fully responsible for his recovery.

23. What is the difference between alternative and complementary medicine?

Alternative and complementary medicines recently have been described as all treatments that traditionally have not been offered to patients in hospital-based oncology practices, including dietary modification and supplementation, herbal products, acupuncture, massage, exercise, and psychological and mind-body therapies. They differ in that alternative therapy is often used instead of standard or "mainstream" medical care, while complementary medicine is used together with standard care. Alternative medicine is often thought of a means of cure, while the goal of complementary medicine is usually improving quality of life through the reduction of physical symptoms and emotional distress while someone undergoes or finishes traditional cancer treatments.

24. What will the doctor think if my loved one uses alternative or complementary techniques? Should I tell the doctor?

Doctors and the medical establishment have been wary of complementary and alternative medicine for a number of reasons. Although some treatments, like traditional Chinese medicine, may represent a centuries-old body of knowledge administered by trained,

Acupuncture
ancient Asian system of therapy that uses long, thin needles to cure disease or relieve symptoms.

Complementary medicine or therapies
healing treatment(s) used together with mainstream, hospital-based medical practice.

Alternative medicine
healing treatment(s) used instead of mainstream, hospital-based healthcare practice.

Managing Medical Treatment and Care

professional practitioners, they have only begun to be evaluated for safety or effectiveness through biomedical research. Sadly, too many alternative and complementary treatments are simply deceptions, the proverbial snake oil, meant to take advantage of the hopes of the uninformed patient. At their worst, they can cause harm to the patient.

Interest in these therapies, however, continues to grow, in part because they help the patient promote a sense of being an active, positive participant in his or her own healing process. As a result, research on complementary and alternative therapies has expanded in recent years. This research, which the government has been sponsoring as well, is examining what—if any—effects these non-traditional therapies have on disease. The questions are whether the particular therapy stops the progression of disease, extends patient survival, or provides a **palliation** (reduction) of symptoms. Research is also examining the risk for side effects and the risk for dangerous interactions when used with conventional treatment.

Palliate

to reduce the severity of, to mitigate. Palliative care focuses on treating the symptoms of disease rather than curing it.

It is the risks of side effects and interactions that are of immediate concern to your doctor. Although doctors may have a skeptical view of complementary and alternative medicine (perhaps due to bias or unfamiliarity with them), it is important that you tell them if the patient is using complementary or alternative medicine so that his or her care is not compromised. Because so many of their patients have been using these therapies, many major cancer centers now offer some of these therapies themselves so that these treatments can be better coordinated and used in conjunction with standard medical care in an integrated fashion.

25. How do I know that my father is eating a healthy diet?

In general, a healthy diet is a balanced diet, one that includes a number of servings from the different food groups: fruits and vegetables, protein, grains, and dairy foods. Of these, fruits and vegetables contain the greatest number of **phytochemicals** that are believed to prevent cancer or improve cancer prognosis. Vegetables and fruits are also low in fat and high in fiber and micronutrients compared with other foods, and are generally better for people's overall health. The key word, however, is balance.

The person with cancer may have to focus on certain nutritional issues according to whether he or she is undergoing treatment, recovering from treatment, trying to prevent recurrence, or living with advanced cancer. During treatment and recovery from treatment, for example, increasing caloric intake is usually emphasized; after surgery, more protein may be recommended to help tissue heal. After certain colon surgeries, for example, a low-fat, low-fiber diet is prescribed during recovery. Sometimes diet can be adjusted to help prevent or control the nausea or diarrhea that results from some kinds of radiation therapy and chemotherapy treatments. And while it does appear that dietary fat plays a role in the incidence of some cancers (particularly colon and prostate), the effectiveness of low-fat diets in preventing recurrence or extending survival has not been definitively proven.

It is important to note that there may be nutritional concerns specifically related to the particular treatment

Phytochemicals
chemicals found in plants.

For a healthy diet, the key word is balance.

a person with cancer is undergoing. Folic acid and vitamin B_6, for example, can interfere with the effectiveness of some chemotherapies. If your father is taking or planning to take nutritional supplements and/or make changes to his normal diet, check with the doctor or nurse to make sure that there is no negative effect either on him or the efficacy of the cancer treatment. The American Cancer Society (ACS) and other resources provide in-depth information about diet during cancer treatment and recovery, including sample menus. See the Appendix on how to order this information.

Mark's comment:

One way to be sure that your friend or family member is eating right is to go shopping for them and, if you have the time and availability, prepare a meal for them once a week. If simple tiredness is preventing them from eating right, then reducing the burden of shopping and cooking might help. If you do cook for them, cook more than they need for one meal, so they can heat up leftovers on days they're too tired to cook for themselves.

26. My mother is losing weight. I am feeling so frustrated. How can I get her to eat more?

Getting her to eat more isn't necessarily the only solution to her weight loss. Check with her doctor to make sure you understand the possible physical reasons for why your mother is losing weight. If she seems to be eating her meals and is still not getting enough calories, you can increase the amount she takes in either by increasing the total amount of food she eats, or by seeing that the food she does eat packs more of a punch calorie-wise.

However, if she is not eating all her meals, try to understand the cause(s). One major reason for eating less is poor appetite. This can be related to nausea or to pain and difficulty chewing or swallowing (usually caused by mouth sores or dryness). The medical team can guide you to the correct medications and treatments for these conditions. If these are not issues, a reduced appetite can be traced to changes in taste and sensitivities, an early feeling of fullness, and/or emotional upset.

There are a number of tips that may help increase your mother's appetite. Try making the atmosphere surrounding meals pleasant and sociable, and avoid making it a chore. Smaller meals, eaten throughout the day, can seem more manageable to finish at a sitting, and may enable her to eat more in total than three large meals. Experiment with seasonings to reduce the ones your mother finds unpleasant, and substitute others she finds more appealing. Light exercise before meals also helps to stimulate the appetite. Have your mother avoid foods and drinks that cause gas and thus lead to an early sensation of being full.

To increase the amount of protein and calories in the food she does eat, adding butter, sour cream, and yogurt to dishes not only helps to boost the number of calories, but also improves their taste. Substituting milk for water in soups, sauces, or in hot cereals can also add calories to her diet, but check with the doctor or dietitian to make sure that the extra calcium or fat will not be a problem. Use nuts, wheat germ, and peanut butter as protein-rich additions to snacks, and encourage your mother to enjoy these snacks throughout the day. Eating high-calorie foods and trying to gain weight can represent a major shift for most people, who for most of their lives tried not to gain, or even lose pounds. It may take time for your mother to shift her way of thinking.

For more tips on how to raise the caloric and nutritional value of your mother's diet, or to look into the possibility of using commercially prepared supplements, check with a dietitian, nurse, or pharmacist. If you are interested in vitamin supplements or medications to further stimulate the appetite, be sure to check with your mother's nurse or doctor before adding them to her diet.

PART THREE

Helping Your Loved One Cope

I feel as though our lives have been out of control since my partner was diagnosed with cancer. How can we regain control of our lives?

I have heard that "positive thinking" can help cure cancer. Does this mean I should discourage my wife from thinking negatively?

How do I help my loved one better manage the emotional "ups" and "downs"?

More...

27. Our lives have been out of control since my partner was diagnosed with cancer. How can we regain some control?

Loss of control is a common feeling for people with cancer. Most aspects of their lives are going to be disrupted, at least temporarily. People with cancer may feel that their own body has turned against them and that body functions that were once automatic may now be less in their control. They may have difficulty with altered bowel movements, appetite and weight change, pain, and/or when surgery and other treatments change their bodies. Attending medical appointments, dealing with insurance, and handling many other issues disrupt usual routines. The side effects of treatment (e.g., nausea, fatigue, and weight changes) may affect their—and your—ability to socialize or participate in usual activities.

These disruptions associated with cancer diagnosis leave some people feeling frustrated and depleted. Try to remind your partner and yourself that many of these disruptions are temporary and will subside. Be aware that concerns about control in some areas sometimes lead a person to believe that *all things* are out of his or her control. This simply is not true. Some ways to help yourself include focusing on what you can control, including engaging in enjoyable activities (either old or new ones), asking for assistance when needed, and learning about other ways that you can help yourself (see Part 4: "Caring for Yourself"). Remember that learning more about the disease, its treatment, and the side effects of treatment can be important steps toward normalizing your life and taking back control. You will know what is expected and when to seek medical attention, making the process seem more in your control and less intimidating.

28. Did stress or depression cause the cancer?

Many people believe that stress, depression, or personal characteristics lead to cancer development and affect its growth. There are books written on the subject, and the media seem to report on this issue frequently. Additionally, this belief is hard to challenge. People want to believe that there is a cause for their loved one's cancer, and they often focus on what is sometimes called the "mind-body connection."

Simply put, *it is very unlikely that stress or depression causes cancer*. Despite research linking stress and/or other emotional reactions to specific changes in people's hormone levels, certain types of immune functioning, and influencing other medical problems such as heart disease, this connection has not been proven for cancer. It is not true that someone "gave himself cancer" by having certain personality characteristics, being depressed, or being stressed.

The few research studies that have shown a relationship between stress or other psychosocial issues and cancer have been limited in scope, have flaws in their research design, and have been widely questioned by specialists in this area. Other researchers have tried to replicate and improve these studies, but so far have failed to find a cause–effect relationship between stress and/or depression and cancer growth or length of survival. Further research is needed to investigate the mind-body connection more fully, and many researchers are focusing on this topic.

We do know, however, that mood and other emotional factors may lead to behaviors that promote health. These behaviors, in turn, may indirectly enhance life expectancy. For example, a person who is enthusiastic about life, enjoys walking several miles a day, and eats balanced meals would be more likely to have regular health check-ups and seek medical attention if something physically didn't feel right. Early intervention may detect cancer at an earlier stage, increasing the chances of effective treatment. Alternatively, a person who is eternally pessimistic and hopeless may postpone important medical tests, such as a colonoscopy to screen for colorectal cancer, or refuse or delay cancer treatment because he erroneously believes that negative outcomes are inevitable. Therefore, delaying medical attention may affect the likelihood that the cancer is treated successfully. If you believe that distress may be affecting your loved one's health-related or medical decisions, discuss this with him or her and suggest speaking with the doctor, or possibly a counselor.

29. I have heard that "positive thinking" can help cure cancer. Does this mean I should discourage my wife from thinking negatively?

Sometimes I don't feel so positive, and the rest of family gets upset with me when I express negative thoughts, such as speculating whether the surgery and treatments actually will work, or sometimes wondering whether it is worth going through all this. Now, I am not only feeling guilty about having negative thoughts because I may be hurting my chances of survival, but I also feel that I am letting my family down.

Jean, age 46, high-school teacher, diagnosed with colon cancer.

One of the most common questions from patients and their family members is about the role of "positive thinking." As discussed in Question 28, research has not yet found a conclusive cause-and-effect relationship between positive thinking, personality characteristics and/or coping styles and cancer development, diagnosis, or prognosis. The relationship between mental events and physical events is not clearly understood. Thinking negatively or positively has not been proven to directly affect cancer growth or to cure cancer.

Sometimes, people believe that thinking positively all the time is necessary. Consequently, they then feel guilty when they cannot perform this impossible task, because they think that they are negatively affecting their health or chances of survival by periodically having a negative attitude. However, it is unrealistic to expect any person to be upbeat all of the time.

Even though positive thinking may not directly affect someone's cancer, many people find that maintaining a hopeful, positive outlook does make them feel better. Positive thinking can help decrease distress, which in turn can make a person better able to handle treatments and possible side effects. People can help themselves through difficult times by viewing life as worth living, seeking enjoyment, connecting with others, and seeing themselves as fighters who will survive. Remember, however, that trying to think positively all the time is simply not possible and can itself cause undue stress.

When a person with cancer expresses negative emotions such as fear and sadness, people around them often will try to support them with quick statements like, "Don't think/feel that way! You'll be OK!" Although the patient indeed may have misconceptions about his or her disease, or inadequate information,

Thinking negatively or positively has not been proven to directly affect cancer growth or to cure cancer.

Helping Your Loved One Cope

statements like these from others can make the person with cancer feel as though he or she is not being heard. The person feels that what he or she says is being devalued and dismissed.

Of course, it is difficult to hear a loved one express negative emotions. However, this may be a necessary step for him or her to come to terms with the diagnosis and the life changes that follow. Allowing your loved one to be truthful may be the most important thing you do as a caregiver.

30. How do I help my loved one better manage the emotional "ups" and "downs"?

Positive coping

techniques of thinking and behaving that help a patient respond to an event or stress more effectively.

Expressing both positive and negative thoughts and emotions is normal. This is as much a concern for you as it is for the person with cancer. You and your loved one can balance your emotions by focusing on the positive in addition to recognizing the unpleasant thoughts. Think of this as **positive coping** and not merely "positive thinking." As your loved one becomes more comfortable with this kind of coping, you too may start to feel more comfortable with him or her expressing a mixture of positive and negative reactions. Being more positive doesn't mean erasing everything negative from your consciousness.

Suppression

trying not to think about something.

Furthermore, **suppressing** negative thoughts and emotions does not work because people tend to think more about the very thing they try to forget. In other words, the more someone resists an emotion or thought, the stronger it may become. It's like trying not to think of a white elephant. The more you try not to think of it, the more often a white elephant pops into your mind.

If you or your loved one finds yourself thinking unpleasant thoughts, first of all, do not judge yourself for thinking them. Take some time to focus on those thoughts to help yourself identify what is truly bothering you. Do you picture a certain image, such as an unpleasant medical procedure? A recurring scenario or a particular worry? Sometimes talking about the unpleasant thoughts is a good way of getting to the heart of the concern, and this can help resolve the problem. If you or your loved one find yourself frequently thinking and/or talking about a particular worry, you may want to take action to help yourself, either by solving the problem (if possible) or seeking help from a mental health professional to help you and your loved one cope better with the problem.

Do not try to radically change your or your loved one's personality if either of you is generally a pessimistic person, since this would be nearly impossible. If you are confused about whether either of you is "thinking properly," need help with positive coping strategies, or would like advice on how to better communicate with each other or other family members, speak to your social worker or another counselor for guidance.

31. After being diagnosed with cancer, my husband had a variety of emotional reactions. Is this normal, or is he going crazy on top of having cancer?

Every individual's reaction to cancer is just that—individual. People have both negative and positive reactions to adversity, including a diagnosis of cancer. These reactions may include the following:

- Asking himself why he got cancer

- Feeling more isolated and alone
- Feeling vulnerable and/or less able to control aspects of his life
- Being less able to concentrate
- Blaming himself for his diagnosis
- Viewing his body and himself differently
- Experiencing changes in relationships with family members and friends
- Redefining life priorities
- Reevaluating spiritual beliefs

Common emotions felt by people who have been diagnosed with cancer include *uncertainty* and *fear* of the future, of pain, of loss, of death; *anger*, either diffuse (general) or directed at particular situations or people; *guilt*, for believing they are responsible for putting their families through their diagnosis, and for "imposing" on others for care and support; and *love* and *gratitude* toward people close to them.

A cancer diagnosis often brings people closer to their loved ones. Many patients tell us that they feel more connected and that they love their families even more than before their diagnosis as a result of reevaluating life's priorities. For many people, priorities change after their diagnosis, allowing them to focus on spending time with their significant others and on their love for one another.

32. Who is at higher risk to experience difficulties in coping with cancer?

Some people go through the entire diagnosis and treatment able to maintain a generally positive outlook, managing the medical care while balancing their daily lives. Anyone, however, may experience difficulty in coping. The following situations or characteristics may increase people's distress:

- Past negative experiences with medical treatments or hospitals
- Recent or unresolved losses (including deaths, divorce, job loss)
- Loss of a family member (or friend) to cancer or personal history of previous cancer diagnosis
- Personal or family history of depression, anxiety, or other psychiatric diagnosis
- History of drug or alcohol abuse
- Initial cancer diagnosis at an advanced stage
- Lack of spirituality, religious views, or meaningful life philosophy
- Particularly stressful lifestyle before diagnosis
- Financial concerns
- Generally pessimistic view toward life, or feeling helpless when faced with life challenges
- Past or current trauma (war combat, or physical or sexual abuse)
- Responsibility for minor children or dependent adults
- Being elderly or disabled and living alone; lack of social supports; being isolated
- Relationship or family difficulties

If you identify one or more of these situations and think that they will increase your loved one's distress, consider being proactive by seeking advice from a social worker or seeking support and guidance from professionals, such as Cancer Care, Inc. (see the Appendix for contact information). By asking for help in the beginning, you may be able to prevent distress from getting worse by learning how to help your loved one manage his or her feelings; this will help you to solve some of the problems interfering with successful coping. Further information about types of support and counseling are discussed in Questions 45 and 47.

33. How do I know if the distress has reached such a level that my loved one needs professional help?

Periodic mood swings and distress are normal for patients and family after a diagnosis of cancer and during treatments. However, these normal reactions may become severe enough for a person to experience symptoms of clinical depression, anxiety disorders such as **phobias** or panic attacks, or other treatable psychological problems. In fact, some researchers estimate that as many as 25% to almost 50% of cancer patients experience clinically significant distress, such as depression. If your loved one feels "down" for more than several consecutive weeks, or if unsettling moods interfere with his or her ability to function in daily life, then contact a doctor or mental health professional to discuss possible ways to get help. If the person has a history of abusing or misusing drugs or alcohol, and/or a psychiatric diagnosis, or even has had episodes of feeling depressed or anxious that have not been officially diagnosed, he or she could be particularly susceptible to depression, anxiety, or the misuse of drugs during the stress of this illness.

Phobia

overwhelming fear of an object, situation, or procedure.

Review the list of symptoms for depression and anxiety in Table 1. This list is not comprehensive, and it is not intended for self-diagnosis. It *is* intended to educate you about the possible symptoms of depression and anxiety

Table 1   Symptoms of depression and anxiety

- Sleep disturbances
- Appetite changes, weight fluctuation
- Little enjoyment of activities that you used to like
- Increased thoughts about death, hopelessness, and sometimes thoughts or plans of suicide
- Feeling fatigued or having little energy
- Being physically slowed down, or the opposite, feeling nervous or restless
- Depressed mood or sadness, tearfulness
- Feeling alone and isolating yourself from others
- Being less able to concentrate or make decisions
- Feeling worthless or guilty
- Uncontrollable or excessive anxiety or worry
- Fear or phobia of a specific situation or event (needles, blood draws, going to hospitals)
- Being more irritable or agitated
- Engaging in compulsive behaviors (e.g., seeking reassurance by repeatedly asking the same questions)
- Feeling muscle tension
- Mentally and emotionally re-experiencing past upsetting events

Derived from *Diagnostic and Statistical Manual of Mental Disorders,* 4th Edition (DSM-IV).

disorders (which can occur simultaneously). There are many other psychological problems that have different symptoms. Sometimes it is hard to distinguish between the physical side effects of certain treatments or symptoms related to the cancer itself and the symptoms of distress. Therefore, if you or your loved one experiences the symptoms listed or others that are not listed, and these symptoms persist for over two weeks, tell your physician and/or other mental health professionals so that they can accurately diagnose and treat so that you or your loved one can start to feel better. Call 911 if anyone is planning suicide or harm to someone else. A description of different types of mental health professionals is provided in Question 47.

34. How do I help my partner manage the stress? The cancer diagnosis, upcoming surgery, and possible chemotherapy and radiation therapy all seem so overwhelming. Where do I begin?

First, identify your partner's past coping techniques. Start by looking back on how he or she has coped with difficult situations in the past. People tend to use the same coping techniques to deal with difficult, but different, situations. Have his or her methods been productive and effective? As long as they weren't negative forms of coping, such as drug or alcohol abuse, overeating or under-eating, or violent behavior, it may be that past coping strategies are still effective now.

Generally speaking, learning about the diagnosis and treatment in advance of the office visit may make particularly stressful situations more manageable. Patients often describe the time before surgery or chemotherapy and radiation therapy as particularly stressful. They play the "hurry up and wait game," which describes the situation of feeling the urgency of getting a definitive diagnosis, establishing treatment and other important aspects of the disease, and then waiting for treatments to begin. They have described the fear that the cancer is still growing in their bodies. Some people may demand radical treatment prematurely as a result of this stress, and this could be an irreversible decision that these people later regret.

Furthermore, patients often misunderstand chemotherapy and radiation therapy, and this misunderstanding can cause extreme fear and dread in some patients. For example, some people assume that they will be very sick (including nausea, diarrhea, and so on), be in pain, and/or lose their hair. True, some patients may experience one or more of these symptoms, but new cancer treatments, and medications that control side effects, enable patients to better tolerate radiation therapy and chemotherapy. Many people experience few or no side effects. Others do experience more side effects, but they continue to maintain an active lifestyle with minor changes to their daily activities.

It can help if you and your partner talk with a former patient whose treatment was similar to your partner's, to pick up some useful tips on how to manage treatments. If the plan is to have chemotherapy or radiation therapy, and your partner is someone who likes to be informed and prepared, you and your partner may consider making a visit to the treatment area(s) before starting treatment in order to familiarize yourself with the environment. Sometimes it helps to actually see the treatment areas. It makes them seem less mysterious and can make it easier to visualize the future. The "unknown" thus becomes more known, which can lessen the degree of fear. Most importantly, speak with your partner's doctor or nurse to get correct information about what to expect from your partner's specific type of treatment, including possible side effects and how to prevent or treat them.

Of course, it may happen that your partner feels frustrated by limitations her body places on her, such as fatigue or other symptoms, during the treatments or after surgery. Remind her to pace herself, and to make adjustments according to how she is feeling. This requires a mental adjustment of how much her body can handle now versus what it could handle before cancer treatment. For example, your partner may enjoy seeing movies but now may not have enough energy to make a trip to the theater. Rent a movie instead and stay at home. She may have only enough energy some nights to watch part of the movie. This is OK. Everyone needs rest to recuperate, and pushing someone past reasonable limits can be counterproductive, resulting in more fatigue and stress.

Another important coping method for many people is using the social support of friends, family, colleagues, or others in their "immediate world." If possible, help your loved one identify one or two people with whom he or she can openly share feelings and fears. Just talking about thoughts, feelings, and concerns is one of the best ways to get things off one's chest, problem solve, and obtain help from others.

35. I've heard that exercise can reduce stress. But won't it use up energy my spouse should use to fight the cancer?

Moderate exercise and activity can help patients combat fatigue and maintain muscle strength.

Yoga

ancient Hindu system of philosophy that employs physical exercise and diet restrictions to control the functioning of the mind and body.

Recent research is showing positive benefits of exercise for people with cancer. Under the supervision of a doctor, moderate exercise and activity can help patients combat fatigue and maintain muscle strength, which can be diminished by surgery and other treatments. Exercise also helps patients to decrease anxiety, reduce feelings of depression, and maintain a positive body image. Some hospitals are incorporating exercise classes, including **yoga**, chair aerobics, and personal training, all facilitated by specially trained experts.

If your spouse is interested, help him by investigating local exercise programs, either through the hospital, a local gym, physical therapist, or community group, and be sure someone who has experience working with people with cancer leads the programs. It is crucial that patients undergo any exercise routine safely to avoid injury and to benefit from the exercise. The cost of such services and programs varies. However, community groups such as senior centers, Gilda's Club, and the American Cancer Society sometimes sponsor exercise activities free of charge.

People also can increase activity in their everyday lives without going to classes or a gym by walking more or taking the stairs at the hospital instead of the elevator, even if they have the energy for just one flight. One patient, who was having a hard time with fatigue due to his chemotherapy and radiation therapy, felt that walking his hallway several times a day kept his body working and helped maintain his mental strength as well. Being active includes fun things too, like going to the mall shopping, walking the dog, or playing with the kids. Doing activities with the patient can allow for quality time together. And, having an exercise partner will be good motivation for both of you, since exercise can be an important part of reducing stress and improving health. Keep it fun!

36. What can help my loved one to relax during treatments and tests?

Relaxation techniques can reduce distress during certain treatments (such as chemotherapy or radiation therapy). Relaxation also has helped people reduce their perception of pain. One can start simply by using self-taught relaxation techniques, such as simple deep breathing techniques, which can be very effective. People with cancer may bring calm music CDs or tapes to treatments or a hospital stay. (Which also may be used to drown out the snoring patient next to them!) To obtain further guidance in using more advanced relaxation techniques, such as **hypnosis** or **progressive relaxation,** you can ask the physician, nurse, or social worker for a referral to licensed practitioners of yoga, massage, relaxation training, hypnosis, reflexology, and other methods of complementary therapies. Some hospitals and private centers provide comprehensive services that can work in conjunction with the medical treatment.

Many books are available describing methods of stress-reduction and relaxation techniques. No matter what you and your partner choose to do, discuss the plan first with the doctor to avoid any complications. For example, some types of **touch therapy,** such as massage, may not be recommended by doctors if a person has cancer **metastases** in his or her bones or certain other conditions. Complementary therapy can begin after it has been approved by the doctor.

As a family member, you can learn to be an effective "relaxation coach" for the patient. We have seen family members learn basic touch therapy, and other relaxation techniques such as guided visualization, that dramatically help the patient cope with pain, nausea, and periods of high distress. You may find using the relaxation techniques for yourself helpful, too.

37. My husband has very little to say about his cancer, other than, "The doctors will take care of it." How do I break through his denial?

"**Denial**" is a loaded word. Many people use the word denial, typically when referring to it as a negative way to cope. However, denial, in fact, can be a useful cop-

Hypnosis

artificially induced trance-like state of consciousness in which the subject is susceptible to suggestion. Used in symptom relief and to reinforce behavioral change.

Progressive relaxation

relaxation technique using deep breathing and muscle control exercises; can also incorporate peaceful music and guided imagery.

Touch therapy

massage or acupressure.

Metastasis

the spread of cancer from the primary (original) tumor to another part of the body.

Denial

a defense mechanism people use to reduce their distress. Can include minimizing the significance of a stressful event, or in the extreme, denying its existence at all.

ing technique, serving as a **defense mechanism** to *temporarily* shield people from their emotions. Denial can help someone to avoid thoughts or emotions that would be too much to handle at one time. Denial can be useful, but when it compromises a person's ability to cope, follow medical advice, or is extreme (to the point where he denies he even has cancer, for instance), it can lead to higher levels of stress. In particular, people who deny a problem are less likely to solve it or ask for help when needed. Give your husband time to come to grips with the situation. If being stoic is normal for him, then he may continue to use this method of coping; it does not necessarily mean that he is "in denial" or that his coping method is a bad thing. For someone like this, being forced to talk about the cancer and feelings may make him feel worse. Be gentle, supportive, and let him come around on his own schedule and in his own way. If his reaction is not typical of his personality, speak with him directly about your perceptions and concerns, and explain how his reduced communication affects your feelings. Initiate the conversation with "When you do this, I feel..." Phrasing it as an "I statement" is less threatening, as it puts the focus on you and your feelings, reducing the likelihood that he will feel blamed, threatened, or attacked.

38. What about God and religion? Will it help to discuss these things now?

Often, people need help answering difficult questions that arise about their spirituality and beliefs—sometimes they may even question long-held beliefs. Many people wonder why they or their family member was diagnosed with cancer, and they speculate about whether God is punishing them, or maybe testing them. These thoughts are common, but they also can

Defense mechanism

a psychological method of protecting oneself from anxiety or high emotional distress.

Helping Your Loved One Cope

Faith and the strength derived from spirituality can be a crucial part of coping with a diagnosis of cancer.

create added anxiety if left unaddressed. Faith and the strength derived from spirituality can be a crucial part of coping with a diagnosis of cancer. If you or your spouse belongs to a religious group, or if you attend services, you may find further support from others in your religious community. Many people with cancer and their families have been comforted by their own prayers and by knowing that others are praying for their recovery. You may choose to meet with a hospital chaplain or use your own spiritual support system to begin to understand your current experiences in the context of your own beliefs. Seeking meaning in your lives, especially in the context of the diagnosis, can be an important part of exploring spirituality. Even if you are not religious or spiritual, you and your partner may have philosophical concerns you may want to discuss with a hospital chaplain or with someone else you trust.

39. After telling my wife she had cancer, one of the first things the doctor suggested was that she stop smoking. She's tried in the past, but it hasn't worked. How can I help her?

It's not easy to give up tobacco use. It's all the more difficult when there is a physical dependency involved. Many people who use tobacco find the drug nicotine to be powerfully addictive. Some smokers can just quit cold turkey; many others, however, have to make numerous attempts before they successfully quit and put the tobacco use behind them once and for all. There are many methods to assist people to quit smoking, however, and your encouragement can be an important part of her support system.

By now, your loved one has probably understood the message that smoking is bad for her, and the sooner she quits, the better. She may not know, however, that no matter how long she might have smoked, quitting now can have real health benefits. Some people assume that after a certain point, it's too late to help, but this is not true. Ask about her thoughts regarding quitting or not quitting, but don't preach or criticize. Rather than trying to provide her with the "correct" information, it's more important to understand, from *her* point of view, her smoking and her difficulty with quitting. Gently ask her what the reasons are for her smoking, and what her barriers are to quitting. After listening to what she has to say, follow up by asking her what she thinks you can do to help.

Being a supportive partner requires you to be non-judgmental. Nagging and confronting the smoker with threats will only undermine your ability to help. Ultimately, it's her decision to make. Being a positive influence—offering praise and encouragement, rewarding her for the progress she makes, however small, helping her to find other ways of relieving the stress that may be causing her to smoke in the first place—is a much better way of showing how much you care for her, whether she quits or not.

Social support is a tremendous asset in helping someone to quit smoking. You can recruit other family members and friends to provide more positive reinforcement for your wife. There are also smoking cessation programs that can provide individual or group-based counseling and support. You can probably find these services at your local major medical center or through such national organizations as the American Cancer Society and the American Lung Association (see the Appendix for contact information).

Nicotine replacement therapy (such as "the patch," nicotine gum, inhalers that look like cigarettes or nasal spray), counseling, and Zyban (a prescription medication) are available and have been shown to improve a person's chances of successfully quitting. Behavioral techniques also can be particularly effective. When a tobacco craving occurs, simply waiting five minutes, drinking a glass of water, or finding another distraction will allow the craving to pass without choosing to smoke a cigarette. Additionally, changing routines that lead to smoking and avoiding "hot spots" for smoking can be tremendously helpful in stopping cravings. For example, if your wife smokes during her morning routine, such as when she's drinking coffee, she can change her morning routine to disrupt the link to smoking (perhaps by having her coffee later in the morning). Or, if she tends to drink in bars or on breaks at work, she can avoid these pressure situations for awhile until she has successfully quit and can better resist temptation.

People often try to quit many times before they are eventually successful.

Keep in mind that people often try to quit many times before they are eventually successful. If your wife tries and then "fails," try to help her see this temporary quitting as a partial success rather than a total failure. Encourage her to try again when she is ready, and since she has had practice quitting before, the next time may be even easier. If she has been hospitalized for awhile and cannot smoke, the admission can be the jump-start to a long-term attempt at quitting. Also, if you also use tobacco (even cigars, pipes, or chewing tobacco), quitting together might give you both the extra support you need.

PART FOUR

Caring for Yourself

Am I getting "burned out"? What are the signs, and how do you prevent caregiver burnout?

What are support groups, and how can they help me? If I decide to try out a group, how do I locate one that is right for me?

Despite the fact that my son was diagnosed with cancer almost two months ago, I constantly think about his cancer and feel down much of the time. What should I do? Would counseling help?

More . . .

40. Lately I seem to think a lot about other bad things that have happened to me in my life. I don't usually dwell on the past. Is something wrong with me now?

Thinking about the past can serve many useful purposes. When things go wrong and life becomes difficult, it's natural to wonder why such things happen and to try to uncover the causes. A normal response is to want to "fix it." Common questions for all of us include: "What did I do wrong? Should I have known something like this could happen? What could I have done differently to avoid this or make it better?"

Revisiting the times when you struggled in your life can be instructive. One way to help yourself is by taking an inventory of the different ways you managed problems before and how well your methods of coping worked. You can apply these past coping methods to your current problems, or develop new ways of dealing that will be better at reducing your distress. For example, previously you may have had another family member who experienced a life-threatening illness (perhaps a parent). Was it helpful at that time to have the involvement and encouragement of other family or friends? Were there any particular questions for the medical team that you wished you had asked, that would have helped to prepare you for what occurred later? What ways did you temporarily distract yourself or take breaks?

Experience is not only a means for us to learn how to do things better, however. It also gives us our sense of who we are as individuals and the meaning of our lives. A life is never all negative or all positive; it's always a combination of both. It's just as necessary to mourn our losses as it is to celebrate our joys and triumphs. But, if you find yourself thinking only about the negative, only about all the losses in your life, it's important to balance that by defining everything good and valuable about yourself and your life as well. Otherwise, you may be practicing an unrealistic, skewed pattern of thought that can contribute to deepening sadness and emotional difficulties. If this is the case, speak with someone whose opinion you value and trust in an effort to regain a balanced perspective. If, on the other hand, you find yourself "stuck," thinking that everything in your life has always been—and always will be—bad or terrible, it is probably time to seek counseling to explore how your past may be influencing the present.

41. Thinking about the future and everything that has to be done—how can I manage this practically?

Focus on one day at a time, one moment at a time, and solving one problem at a time. Try to move beyond thinking about the past, "what-ifs," and "why's." Instead, focus on the present and about how you and your partner are going to cope with the current problems, here and now. In other words, *be in the moment.* If you are feeling happy and calm, allow yourself to sit and enjoy this feeling. Whenever you are feeling distressed, identify what you are experiencing physically and emotionally. This will help you begin to focus on identifying the problem and to help solve it. By focusing on the issue at hand, you may then be able to formulate a plan that can reduce feelings of hopelessness and helplessness.

If you are already on "emotional overload," first step back a moment and identify what you were thinking about before you felt overwhelmed. Were you worrying about all the doctor appointments or things you have to do but are not able to given time or other constraints? Second, identify your feelings. For example, do you feel regret or frustration at not being able to do what you want or believe you need to do? Next, problem solve by prioritizing your commitments according to their importance and according to other factors, such as your energy levels and other limits. Can someone else help you? By breaking down surmounting obligations, you will take control, be less overwhelmed, and reduce negative feelings.

Tip: Take out a pen and paper, and make a list of priorities. Circle or mark some problems that you can solve now. Solving a few smaller problems first will help you feel that you are making some concrete steps toward accomplishing your goals.

42. Am I getting "burned out"? What are the signs, and how do you prevent caregiver burnout?

The chronic stresses of caregiving—being responsible and providing care for another person while adjusting your own life according to that person's needs—can leave you feeling overburdened, resentful, and depressed. Unless these stresses are relieved, or you find ways replenish your emotional and physical reserves, you as a caregiver might wind up burned out. Burnout can include being exhausted, feeling hopeless about the future, and no longer caring about what happens either to yourself or your loved one.

Warning signs of burnout include:

• Irritability and a low tolerance for frustration

- Constant exhaustion
- Problems sleeping
- Decreased interest in activities you used to enjoy
- Social isolation
- Recurring feelings of guilt and/or anxiety

If you think you are at risk for burnout, one of the first things you should do is acknowledge the toll the tasks of caregiving are exacting from you and to give yourself permission to look after your own needs. It is essential that in addition to focusing on the patient's needs, you make your own needs a priority as well. Take time out for yourself, away from the cancer and the hospital. Ask another family member/caregiver or friend to step in to help, if needed. If you do not take care of yourself, you will not be at your best for the patient.

If you are having problems managing your stress levels, find a professional to talk to or find a family/caregiver support group in your area. You may choose to talk to your loved one with cancer or someone else, such as a good friend, family member, or maybe a family member of another patient who is going through similar experiences. You can also meet other family members at various medical appointment waiting rooms or other places, such as support groups.

The following suggestions also might help make caregiving more manageable and prevent burnout.

- Learn to delegate responsibility to others and draw upon people outside the household for help.
- Recognize your limits and learn to say no to things you cannot be responsible for.
- Nourish yourself physically by maintaining a proper diet and exercising.

If you do not take care of yourself, you will not be at your best for the patient.

- Take care of your emotions by accepting and expressing even your negative feelings.
- If you are religious or spiritual, remember to replenish yourself spiritually to find strength through your connection with nature, religion, or some other faith-based system of meaning.

43. I have not seen my friends for weeks. Sometimes I feel that I just need to get away from the hospital, doctors, and the cancer for awhile. How can I do this without feeling too guilty?

Spending time with your friends and supportive family members is one of the most important buffers against stress for caregivers of people with cancer. And getting away from the hospital and cancer for a while is a very important part of taking care of yourself and avoiding burnout. However, feeling conflicted about being there for the patient versus focusing on your own needs is common among family members whom we see. Do you feel guilty? If so, why?

Family members often tell us that they feel guilty about having fun when their loved one is sick with cancer. Or, they feel that if they leave, something bad will happen, and it will be their fault. The fact is, when asked, patients usually would rather see their family members taking breaks. It not only gives them time to themselves, but also somewhat relieves their own guilt that they are constantly a burden to others. Good feelings are "contagious." If you feel better, the patient might brighten up, too.

If you are having trouble pulling yourself away to spend time with members of your support network, start slowly. Begin by asking your friends to come over to your home, or meet them someplace for coffee near your home or the hospital. Get a cell phone, if needed, and check in with your loved one while you are away. If you want, talk to your friends about how you feel. Or, just use the time to distract yourself by talking about their lives or other topics for awhile. The patient may appreciate some time alone, too. On some occasions, bring your loved one with you to do something fun, as long as the doctor says it's OK. This way you will be spending time with him or her while both of you have a good time.

44. Even though I feel overwhelmed, I don't think that it's right to think of my needs right now. Shouldn't I be doing everything possible to help the patient?

In times of crisis and great distress, we are often able to summon tremendous reserves of strength and endurance to protect and support our loved ones who are hurt or suffering. It's natural to want to devote every ounce of energy to this task, in the hope of some benefit to our loved one, regardless of the physical, emotional, or spiritual toll on ourselves. "After all," we believe, "this is what I have to do now, at whatever cost. I'll have time later on to deal with the consequences."

The problem is, if you're pushing yourself too hard and too long, you may be compromising your ability to support the patient, both now and in the future. Pushing your limits can drain energy and increase stress.

You may also neglect your own health under such circumstances. For example, we have seen many caregivers postpone their own medical care out of feeling obligated to spend all their time with person with cancer. If you get sick, won't this affect the care you are able to provide to the patient? If your emotions are threatening to unravel, how helpful can you be to a patient who's trying to calmly chart a course through treatment? It is very important that you attend to your own medical, physical, and psychological needs.

Furthermore, a caregiver may not see that other family members feel neglected or overlooked because all of his or her attention and energy is devoted to the patient. For example, if you have children, the care you provide them may change in the face of new responsibilities in caring for the person with cancer. Be sure that other people dependent on you are well cared for and safe.

Although it's difficult, it's sometimes necessary to take a step back and examine what you are doing for the patient, and why. Providing too much care, even out of love, is detrimental when it undermines the confidence and ability of patients to perform the tasks they are capable of doing themselves. Even when the care is necessary, is it truly required that you alone have to provide it? For many reasons, sometimes caregivers have difficulty letting others help them assist the patient. This is often not reasonable or sustainable, depending on the level of assistance the patient needs.

Of course, there are some barriers in getting help from family, friends, or healthcare professionals.

Other family members may have jobs and/or their own families to care for; insurance will not cover enough hours for help at home, and there is no money to pay for private care. Address these problems with the help of a social worker or whomever you feel comfortable with as a problem-solving partner. But understand, too, that respecting your own needs does not necessarily mean doing less for your loved one. Sacrifice is not the same as martyrdom. By remembering to protect and nurture yourself, you will be that much stronger and better equipped emotionally and physically to help your loved one through hard times.

Home care options are discussed in Part Six and sources of financial assistance are discussed in Part Seven of this book.

45. What are support groups and how can they help me? If I decide to try out a group, how do I locate one right for me?

People with cancer and their family members often find that talking to other people who are also affected by cancer helps them understand that they are not alone. They may learn new ways of coping and be relieved to be able to discuss their concerns openly with someone who has had similar experiences and understands.

There are different types of support groups. Some agencies, such as Cancer Care, Inc., offer traditional groups as well as innovative groups that are conducted on the Internet and on the telephone. These latter two types of groups are particularly helpful to people who are not comfortable meeting many new people, for those who simply do not feel well enough to travel from their homes, and for those who live too far away from group meetings.

Professionals facilitate some groups, while cancer survivor volunteers or family members of patients (for groups intended for family) lead other groups. **Therapy groups** are intended to treat a specific psychological problem, such as clinical depression, and are usually led by a mental health professional. **Support groups** focus on sharing experiences, providing emotional support to people as well as helping to reduce distress and relieve isolation. **Educational groups**, on the other hand, are used to provide information to a large group of people, such as different coping techniques, relaxation training, and management of medical issues. This kind of group focuses less on people sharing their feelings and may be good for those who do not want to attend a traditional support group, but would still benefit from interaction with others. Support and education-focused groups can be led by a variety of professionals and/or survivor volunteers. For help locating support groups, speak with your medical team and/or social worker, or consult our resource list at the back of this book. The American Cancer Society can be particularly helpful in directing you to local groups.

Questions to ask when investigating a group:

1. Does a professional lead this group? Or does a volunteer facilitate it?
2. Do I have to commit to a certain number of sessions?

Therapy groups

group counseling to treat a specific therapeutic issue (i.e., depression, anxiety, etc.) led by a mental health professional.

Support groups

a gathering that is focused on sharing experiences, providing emotional support and relieving the sense of isolation. May be led by social workers or trained cancer survivor volunteers.

Educational groups

a gathering of people where information is presented on a range of topics (i.e., coping techniques, relaxation methods, management of medical issues).

3. What date does the group start? How long is each session?

4. Where does the group meet, and may I have directions to the meeting?

5. Is there a cost to attend this group? If so, do you accept my insurance?

6. What topics are covered? Is this a group for people with specific problems (e.g., depression, anxiety, family concerns)?

7. Does this group focus on a specific cancer diagnosis?

8. Are family members/caregivers invited to attend?

46. I am not really interested in attending a group or talking with a bunch of people about my caregiver concerns. Where do I find other caregivers with whom I can talk one-on-one?

Buddy programs exist that link fellow caregivers together for added emotional support and information exchange, ranging from basic advice to more complex problems, such as coping with a new diagnosis. Some useful resources are the National Family Caregivers Association, the American Cancer Society, Cancer Care, Inc., and other resources discussed in the Appendix. Informally, you may meet fellow caregivers at hospital appointments or waiting rooms. Buddy programs are available for patients as well. These cancer survivor volunteers can suggest strategies for your loved one about how to get through surgery, chemotherapy and/or radiation therapy, how to deal with common frustrations of interfacing with the

Caring for Yourself

medical system, and so on. Most importantly, survivor volunteers provide hope to people who are currently battling cancer. Many hospitals and doctors have formal and informal ways of connecting you with cancer survivors and caregivers for support. Your doctor, nurse, or social worker may have suggestions on finding a cancer survivor, or a person going through similar challenges, with whom your loved one can meet, in addition to the community agencies mentioned above.

47. Despite the fact that my son was diagnosed with cancer almost two months ago, I constantly think about his cancer and feel down much of the time. What should I do? Would counseling help?

Despite using adaptive coping skills, many people still find that further guidance is helpful. A good place to start finding help is the medical team (e.g., the doctor, nurse, social worker, or chaplain). For patients themselves, pain and other physical symptoms may be alleviated, making them feel less down or preoccupied. Family members may also respond with distress if their loved one is suffering. Even if physical symptoms are not a contributor, people may feel better after a conversation about their thoughts and feelings, particularly because feeling depressed and anxious is common among family members. *You may feel relieved to know that others have experienced similar feelings.* However, if you still feel that you would like further help managing your thoughts and feelings or if you think you may be suffering from more serious forms of depression or anxiety (see Question 33), you may want to explore additional methods of getting support. Many places provide support and counseling. Meet with your hospital social worker or contact your local chapter of the American Cancer Society to point you in the right direction. If your insurance company covers counseling, review their list of mental health professionals to find an appropriate professional to help.

Many people find that counseling (or psychotherapy) helps them to deal with the emotional aspects of having a cancer diagnosis in the family. Professionals are trained to help people feel their best, both psychologically and emotionally. Below is a brief list of the most common mental health professionals.

Licensed Clinical Social Workers (commonly "CSW" or "LCSW"): Trained clinicians, usually with at least a master's degree (MSW, MSSW, DSW, PhD) and additional training or expertise in their specialty. Clinical social workers practice in a variety of settings, including hospitals, counseling or mental health centers, and private practice. Depending on their expertise, they are able to diagnose and treat psychological problems using counseling. They are also trained in more general counseling to help patients and family members through difficult time periods, with or without an exact psychological diagnosis.

Licensed practical nurse (LPN)

has completed a two-year degree in nursing; often involved with hands-on patient care.

Psychologists: Usually have a PhD or a PsyD. Psychologists can also diagnose and treat psychological issues and are usually trained in a specific theory of therapy (e.g., psychodynamic, cognitive/behavioral). Ask a psychologist you are considering as a prospective therapist to explain his or her theoretical orientation and how it may help. Neither psychologists nor social workers can prescribe medications, but they can refer you to a medical doctor (e.g., a primary physician or a psychiatrist), who can evaluate the need for medications to treat depression, anxiety, or other mental health problems.

Psychiatrists: Medical doctors (MDs) who specialize in diagnosing and treating psychiatric disorders by prescribing medications and/or providing psychotherapy. Their area of expertise is determining the possible physiological bases of mental disorders.

Other mental health professionals: Psychiatric nurses, master's-level counselors, pastoral counselors, alternative/complementary medicine practitioners, and other mental health professionals can also provide certain types of counseling and anxiety-reduction techniques. As with choosing any professional, be sure to investigate their qualifications and experience and how their expertise meshes with your needs.

Important Note: If you are thinking about harming yourself or another person, or have plans to attempt suicide, call 911.

Questions to ask a mental health professional:

1. What is your training, and are you licensed to practice in this state?
2. Do you have experience helping people with cancer or family members of people with cancer?
3. What do you charge? Do you accept our insurance policy?
4. How often and where can I be seen (e.g., in a private office, in the hospital)?

5. What do I do about an after-hours emergency? Whom should we call?

6. Do you specialize in family counseling?

48. Should I consider using medications to help my depression and anxiety?

Medications are helpful to some people suffering from depression, anxiety, and high levels of distress. Depression and anxiety involve physiological changes in the brain and can be helped with medications such as anti-depressants and anti-anxiety prescriptions.

Sometimes people are reluctant to take such medication because they are afraid that it means that they are weak or unbalanced, or that their doctor will treat them differently. Keep in mind that medications are concrete means to address specific medical problems for which they are prescribed. They are meant to make the people who take them more comfortable and in control, not to label or to judge them. Taking a prescription to reduce distress does not mean that someone is going crazy. Some people are hesitant to try these medications because of the stigma they believe is attached; many of these people who later take the medications wonder why they waited so long. They feel so much better and are better able to cope and enjoy life. Often these medications are additionally effective when combined with counseling and/or group support.

Taking a prescription to reduce distress does not mean that someone is going crazy.

Although drug therapy can be helpful, these medications are not for everyone. They are not magic pills that will take away all problems; the problems will still exist, but the medications may make them easier to

Caring for Yourself

manage. You need to make the right decision for you. In addition, these medications sometimes take several weeks to start working and may produce side effects; you should discuss the pros and cons of each medicine with your doctor. Sometimes people have to try different types of medication to find the one that works the best. Any physician, such as a primary doctor, can prescribe such medicines for his or her patients; however, it is worth considering an initial evaluation and/or regular follow-up with a psychiatrist. All of this holds true for your loved one as well. If his or her distress is high, consider talking to the doctor about an evaluation for medications or getting a referral to a psychiatrist.

PART FIVE

Relationship and Family Issues

How can I be "strong" and supportive with my spouse while continuing to cope with my own reactions to this diagnosis?

I feel that my husband and I are growing apart since his cancer diagnosis. Why is this happening?

The doctor told me some news about my mother's cancer; should I tell her? Wouldn't it be better not to tell her and avoid upsetting her?

How do we tell the children about the cancer?

More . . .

49. Why is this so frustrating for the both of us?

A person with cancer may experience a number of changes that can cause negative feelings. Caregivers too can be confronted with numerous changes and may have to learn to live with unexpected limitations in their lives. Frustration builds in various ways. Sometimes the problems are minor, but occur frequently, perhaps on a daily basis. Sometimes the problems are major and are the foundation for longer-term changes. These changes may then drive people to alter hopes and plans for the future.

A great deal of frustration from many family members we interview arises from the feeling that change has been imposed upon them without a choice. People naturally wish that none of this ever happened and that they and their loved ones could go back to the way things were before. Facing up to reality, however, doesn't mean fatalistically resigning themselves to the way things are now. Maybe there isn't a magic bullet—at least not now—to solve the most pressing problems, whether it's finding a cure for their loved one's disease or finding the money to pay for all the prescriptions. But what people can control, or at least try to control, is how they respond—emotionally and practically—to life's events. People are always choosing one path over another, and through these choices will retain or regain a sense of hope and purpose. Managing frustration is discussed in Question 51.

50. How do I get away from feeling that the cancer is our entire life?

In the beginning, a diagnosis can reasonably consume a lot of time and energy. After the initial crisis and treatment decisions are made, it is important to allow other aspects of your lives to regain importance. Granted, if a future crisis arises, less urgent things are put on the back shelf—but it is important to keep life as normal as possible. For example, you can also identify some people as "fun activity partners," meaning people that you can just be with, without necessarily talking about the cancer. Go to the movies, go out to dinner, or play golf with these people. Identify other supporters and good distractions in your life, such as attending religious services, going to work, spending time with your family and friends, or taking up a new hobby or class. Do small things for yourself, like buying something fun and spontaneous—a CD from a completely new artist, or a new electronic gadget, maybe even a gossip magazine; your loved one may want to do the same. Ask yourselves what you love in your lives and what you enjoy the most. After you identify these things, do them. Now. Live life! Tell yourselves, "We are fighting for life, so let's take time to enjoy the very thing we are fighting for."

Do small things for yourself.

Despite the seriousness of their cancer diagnosis, many patients and their family members find that humor is crucial to feeling more normal again. Do not forget to laugh. More importantly, do not forget how to laugh. Humor and laughter can defuse tense situations and can be great stress relievers. Find humor and laughter in different places: identify a particularly funny person in your life and spend time with him or her, go to a comedy movie, watch humorous cartoons, read a book from the humor section of the library, or even go to a live comedy show. If you find it hard to do such things, do still try them, and remember to focus on the moment as much as you can. It will help you enjoy the jokes and laugh, lighten your mood, and take your mind off the more serious things for awhile.

Table 2   Tips for managing stress and better coping

- Learn more about the diagnosis and treatments.
- Identify and evaluate past coping techniques: Did they work in the past? Will they work again?
- Utilize the support of friends, family, and colleagues.
- "Be in the moment." Focus on the here and now.
- Adjust yourself to new limits.
- Exercise and be active.
- Find ways to relax.
- Live your life, remember to laugh, and maintain hope.

And no matter what comes your way, try to maintain hope. Hope for the things you feel are vital in your life. Many people hope for doing something special they have planned with family and friends. Others find hope in spiritual and religious realms. Identify what you and your partner hope for, even though this may change over time. Keep this thing in mind because it will help you to remember what you are living for. Table 2 provides some helpful tips.

Mark's comment:

Even during treatment, patients are still people who have lives. During treatment or after treatment, if they really want to live their life, then let them—don't try to wrap them in bubble wrap to protect them. If they want to go sky diving, pay for it! If they want to go skiing, let them—and a new set of skis is always a great gift. The only thing you should insist upon is that when they go off skiing, they need to at least let you know they're going so you don't get worried by their sudden disappearance (which is what my mother did to me and my sister—scared us silly, because we had no idea where she'd gone!). Encourage them to spend their money—even if it is your inheritance; they deserve it.

Oh yeah, and if they feel like buying a Crown Vic police interceptor…like my mother did…just know that it's a very fast car!

51. With the doctor's appointments, the chemotherapy, and all the changes in our lives, both my husband and I seem to "blow up" at the smallest thing. How do we handle this?

Sometimes fluctuations in mood can result in "blow-ups." This may be bickering with loved ones, overreacting to daily hassles (e.g., traffic, your child spilling something, a jar not opening), and just yelling, feeling very angry, or crying abruptly for "no reason." Most people do not have full insight into how their daily levels of stress, or distress, contribute to such behaviors. Think of stress as cumulative. It has a way of adding up. And this build-up of stress can make people react more strongly to a situation than they would have otherwise. Sometimes the situations do not seem particularly upsetting on the surface, but they bring out a strong emotional response.

Jack, a businessman, age 57, initially met with his hospital social worker to get help reducing his "hidden" stress. He said,

I thought that I was dealing with my cancer well—I did not let it get me down and I did not ever cry. I went through a lot, though. I had some complications after surgery, and then I found out that I needed chemo. After I started back to work and taking chemo once a week, I started to feel a little more "edgy," is how I describe it; I was even losing sleep. However, I thought that I was still doing OK. That is, until I found myself getting really annoyed at small things. And I knew that I wasn't doing "OK" when I snapped at my young granddaughter for spilling her juice. This was totally out of character for me. I guess that my feelings were just building up, and they did come out, but not in a good way.

Jack later talked about how he really felt after his diagnosis and through his surgery and chemotherapy. Jack used denial to protect himself from overwhelming emotions at the time of his initial diagnosis when he was making important treatment decisions and when the reality of his cancer diagnosis did not yet seem real to him. However, his use of denial did not work well for him over the long haul, when the reality sank in and his suppressed emotions erupted.

He felt angry at having cancer, overwhelmed by the complications, treatment, and other responsibilities, and he felt guilty for having put his family through his medical problems. He believed that he was the provider and that he was not supposed to be the dependent one. He tried to maintain the "strong but silent" image to others. However, the pressure finally caught up with him, and his "trigger" happened to be his grandchild's accidental spill.

If you and your loved one release emotions in a similar way, you may find stress-reduction counseling helpful, as well as other forms of counseling. Jack needed to meet with his social worker only a couple of times to gain insight into the role that stress and his feelings played in his life. He learned new coping techniques, which helped him gain better control over his reactions to these feelings. He also learned to focus on his love for his family and to use positive coping methods (see Questions 30 and 34) to help him focus on the good things in his life that helped deflect his reactions to the negative experiences.

For some people, however, the management of anger or other potentially caustic emotions is a problem they have tried to deal with all their life. Although relaxation techniques and taking **time-outs** (i.e., actually removing yourself from the emotion-provoking person or situation) can be effective stop-gap measures, longer-term coping may require developing a better understanding of your emotions, and learning how to express them appropriately. People who are perpetually quick to anger may be that way because of certain patterns of thought that lead to emotional meltdowns. They often turn the smallest problem into catastrophes, or take a single event or comment and generalize it for the person or the situation as a whole ("She forgot to call...she doesn't care what happens to me...nobody is helping me at all.")

Time-out

a coping strategy of removing oneself from an emotion-producing person or situation for a short period of time.

In this case, repetitive talking about negative feelings or "venting" your negative emotions may make the problem worse. Without correction, you may be reinforcing anger-provoking patterns of thought and making them all the more powerful. Problem-solving, better communication, and other coping methods may help, but if your negative emotions really seem to be getting the better of you, speak with a mental health professional to discuss counseling. Counseling can be very effective at helping reduce "blow ups."

52. How can I be "strong" and supportive with my spouse while continuing to cope with my own reactions to this diagnosis?

After his wife was diagnosed with cancer, one husband said, "I feel like I am a passenger in a car on a dangerous, icy road. My wife is driving, and she is in ultimately in control of crucial decisions that will affect both of us, and I am fearful of what will happen." Just as patients feel a loss of control when they are diagnosed with a medical illness, caregivers also often feel a loss of control. As a spouse, you are an observer of what is happening, but you are also profoundly affected by your partner's reactions and decisions.

You probably share a large burden of the caregiving responsibilities. Loved ones report periodically feeling helpless and concerned that, no matter how hard they try, they cannot do enough. You may experience feelings similar to that of the patient, such as depression, sadness, anxiety, and fear. Your life will be disrupted, so understand that these adjustments represent significant changes and allow yourself time to come to grips with them. As you are coping with your own reactions to the diagnosis of your loved one, you are also being expected to perform functions that may be new to you.

These changes can cause discord between you and your spouse, particularly if you are not prepared to talk about these issues as they arise or if you have had relationship problems before the diagnosis of cancer. For many couples, communication could use fine-tuning, even before a diagnosis of cancer. If you need some direction on how to begin more open communication about your spouse's diagnosis, start by asking your partner questions about how he or she is feeling (both physically and emotionally), and how you can help. For example, you may ask:

- How are you holding up?
- Tell me, what is this really like for you?
- I notice that you have been quiet lately. Do you mind telling me what you are thinking about?
- I will try to be here for you any way I can. Could you give me some pointers on ways I can help?

You may want to express your own concerns and feelings to your spouse also. Couples often want to protect each other from their feelings, and in essence, put up an emotional wall. If you take the lead, your spouse may feel that it is OK to share as well. However, remember that you do not need to share everything all the time, particularly if you are not comfortable talking about your feelings. Find what works for you—do not force yourself, or your spouse, to talk.

In addition to communicating feelings and needs, you may consider the following suggestions for how to help your partner, depending on how he or she is feeling:

When communicating feelings and needs, find what works for you.

- Try not to let the topic of cancer dominate all conversation. Talk about other things.
- Live life with your spouse. Do enjoyable activities together.
- Buy a thoughtful gift as a token of your feelings. A note tucked in a pocket can be an unexpected reminder that you are thinking about your partner.

- If he or she is agreeable, take on the "public relations" role by communicating to other people how your spouse is doing.
- Touch your spouse. Touch is an important part of intimacy and reassurance, particularly when words are not enough. Touch is also calming.
- Allow your spouse to feel what he or she is feeling. If your spouse is feeling down, ask why he or she is feeling that way, instead of trying to "fix" the problem immediately or pressuring your spouse to be more positive.
- Do gently remind your spouse about positive aspects of life, such as people who love him or her, or upcoming enjoyable events, like a wedding or party.
- Help your spouse feel less dependent and more in control. Reassure your spouse that you are fulfilling your role as caregiver out of love, and try to help your spouse maintain as much control as possible by continuing to participate in household decisions, making social plans, or doing other activities independently according to how he or she is feeling.

Tip: If you are interested in improving communication, keep in mind that "forcing" your spouse to talk, or suddenly changing your methods of communication, may not bring about the intended result of better communication. Instead, try asking open-ended questions and listen to what your spouse says. An open-ended question is one that has to be answered with more than a simple yes or no. It invites the respondent to share or explain his or her thoughts. Wait for the answer. Some people need time to gather their thoughts before expressing them. Listening is just as important as talking (sometimes even more so!).

53. Am I a spouse, or a caregiver?

The simple answer is that you are both spouse and caregiver. Unexpected illness and disability make many couples reexamine their relationships and how they view their respective roles. While they may have previously expected to regard each other, at least ideally, as equal partners, the practical and emotional dictates of caregiving—and the often ambiguous question of who is in control—can alter roles in the relationship between spousal partners, leading to confusion and tension.

People have very different expectations about their roles as spouse, caregiver, or care recipient based on their family history, cultural background, or personal beliefs. While there may be no way to define the ideal relationship for you and your spouse, there are recommendations we can offer to help make the relationship work more effectively.

The way to begin is to have a discussion with each other about how you currently view your roles, and particularly, the boundaries and limits of your respective positions as caregiver and care recipient. Too often, the "well" partner tries to "do it all," repressing his or her own needs in the process, and often forgoing the hopes and plans he or she may have had for the future. If there is a sense of entitlement on the part of the care recipient, fixed in the role of the "sick spouse," this can contribute to feelings of resentment that build over time. Knowing what you and your spouse expect of each other, and then sensitively setting limits, can help reduce the guilt the caregiver may have over "not doing enough" as well as the guilt the care recipient may feel for being a burden and asking for too much.

For example, one spouse, John, felt very uncomfortable assisting his wife to the bathroom during her hospital stay. He felt even more embarrassed when she had "accidents" in her bed when he could not get her up in time. He told us that he felt guilty for his reactions, thinking that he should be able to help his wife in every way. He explained that he had never seen his wife doing her "private bathroom things" in the past, and subsequent discussion with his wife unearthed that she was also embarrassed by her body functions in John's presence. A solution was reached that the spouse would call the nursing aide or his daughter (who was more comfortable assisting in such intimate things) to assist. In the end, John and his wife felt more comfortable by setting some limits to the practical care he provided and making alternative arrangements.

There may be times when rigidity on one or both sides causes communication to become strained. You, for example, would like to turn over some of your caregiving duties to a home attendant, but your spouse refuses to let strangers come into the home. After addressing each other's concerns, it may be necessary to negotiate a compromise position—perhaps getting another family member or a friend to help, or hiring someone to help for a few hours each day or week. Although you want to help your partner to regain a sense of control over his or her life (which may be reduced when faced with illness), this should not come at the cost of surrendering control over your own life. Legitimizing both partner's needs, and then trying to maintain autonomy and flexibility in performing your roles are key strategies for preventing the challenges of caregiving from permanently undermining your relationship.

54. I feel that my husband and I are growing apart since his cancer diagnosis. Why is this happening?

This is a hard question to answer without understanding much about a couple's relationship before the cancer diagnosis. However, cancer is a huge stress on individuals, families, and couples, and this stress can strain even the closest relationships. A primary contributor to emotional distance is blocked communication. A common reaction we see among patient and family alike is a wish to protect the other from unpleasant reactions or feelings. Sometimes, holding back thoughts or emotions is appropriate. However, if this becomes a pattern and these reactions are never discussed, holding back from telling your partner may sometimes seem like keeping a secret.

We have found that if patients and their partners start talking more openly about their fears, emotions, and questions, they often find they have a better understanding of where the other person is coming from, which can make people feel more connected to each other. Discussing feelings or the topic of cancer is difficult, even for the most expressive people. Remember, however, that displaying emotions, even tears, can bring people closer together. Good support is one of the most important parts of positive coping.

Often, reduced intimacy occurs after a cancer diagnosis, and this can contribute to the belief that you are growing apart. This feeling can stem from less effective communication, as stated above, but also from stress, changes in a patient's body image, and side effects of

Displaying emotions, even tears, can bring people closer together.

cancer treatment (such as fatigue, nausea, recuperation from surgery). Part of maintaining or improving communication also starts with the physical connection you and your spouse share. If sexual relations were an important part of your pre-cancer relationship and are not now, you may want to alter how both of you react physically to one another. For example, affection shown by hugs, kisses, and touches may be reassuring to the patient, and to you. As the initial shock of the diagnosis passes, you may find that new ways of physical communication will transform into a sexual connection. Couples also tell us that their sex lives fluctuate, depending on their stress levels. This is normal. When people are preoccupied, sex may be the furthest thing from their minds. For others, it is the best stress-reliever!

55. What techniques can I use to deal with sexual changes associated with cancer?

As a person moves beyond the initial phase of diagnosis and making treatment decisions, questions regarding other aspects of the person's life become increasingly important. Often, such concerns include intimacy, sexuality, and sexual side effects during and after diagnosis and treatment. For some people, however, sex is a difficult topic to talk about, both with their partners and with the medical team. Nonetheless, open communication can be an important factor in maintaining or regaining your sexuality.

Patients having surgery may experience a decrease in sex drive before surgery because they may be preoccupied with the upcoming treatment and, similarly, during the recuperation period. After surgery and during other treatments, they may experience body changes. These include adjusting to scars, removal of body parts (such as a **mastectomy**), or functions altered due to some types of treatments. Depending on the type of treatment, different varieties of sexual problems can result. Some people feel embarrassed about these changes to their bodies, particularly soon after surgery or medical treatment. With time, they can become accustomed to possible body changes, particularly with assistance from medical professionals and by discussing their concerns with the team and their partners. For example, once an incision has healed, it will not be hurt by touching or intimate activity.

If your partner is experiencing sexual changes, and these changes are significantly affecting both of you, this may be a good time to think creatively about sex and intimacy. Touching, caressing, oral and finger stimulation, and use of sexual paraphernalia are sometimes as arousing and stimulating as traditional sexual intercourse (or more so for some people). As you start to experiment, you may find new ways of pleasing your partner and new activities that you enjoy, too. Often, couples experience resurgence in loving feelings toward one another when they are faced with cancer. Focus on these feelings during lovemaking and sexual practice.

As a sexual partner, you may sometimes be in conflict about whether to initiate sexual contact with the patient. Some significant others have avoided any and all mention of sex for fear of offending the patient. We have heard spouses say they feel guilty for having sexual desires while their loved one is ill. Avoiding healthy sexual expression may not be healthy for your

Mastectomy
surgical removal of the breast.

Relationship and Family Issues

95

relationship, particularly if it was an important part of your lives before the cancer. Sexual desire is a healthy, natural aspect of human existence. Talk about your feelings with your partner. Perhaps your desire is very flattering even though he or she may not be feeling particularly physically desirable. If sexual expression is not possible, for any reason, do not push the issue. Show your love by touch and words until the patient is ready.

Patients may be particularly sensitive to initiating intimate relationships with new partners. Beginning sexual expression will take time, and each situation is different. Patients and their partners should listen to themselves and follow their instincts. Also, keep in mind that sexual adjustment, under any circumstance, starts with being informed and with learning good communication skills. .

If you and your loved one continue to have questions or experience problems, you may want to contact a physician or a therapist who specializes in treating sexual issues. Prescription treatments are available to help with maintaining erection or lubricants for improving vaginal lubrication. Preventive measures, such as using vaginal dilators for women undergoing radiation therapy to the pelvic region (which can make the vaginal walls constrict), or surgical procedures, such as reconstruction, may be possible also for some types of sexual dysfunction.

56. We want to have children in the future. Is this possible after cancer?

If you and your partner are thinking about having children after his or her treatment for cancer, talk with the oncology physician as soon as possible. Sometimes radiation therapy, chemotherapy, and certain surgeries can cause infertility for both men and women. To be successful, it is often crucial that steps are taken before treatment for most kinds of alternative fertility options for cancer patients, such as sperm-banking or harvesting eggs. New options are also available, particularly for women, such as preservation of ovarian tissue removed before treatment which can later be implanted into the body after cancer therapy is finished. Eggs are then harvested and fertilized, with the hope of creating embryos. State-of-the-art research is being conducted assessing methods of preserving fertility among cancer survivors at the Center for Reproductive Medicine and Infertility in New York City (see the Appendix for contact information).

In addition to exploring the medical and technology options, also be sure to investigate insurance coverage and the costs associated with such fertility treatments. There are now organizations advocating for better insurance coverage and possible financial assistance to young adult cancer patients for fertility treatments, such as Fertilehope (see the Appendix for contact information).

57. The doctor told me some news about my mother's cancer; should I tell her? Wouldn't it be better not to tell her and avoid upsetting her?

Mark's comment:

If the doctor is telling you things that he isn't telling his patient, I feel that you should FIRE HIM. It is the doctor's responsibility to talk honestly with his patient, and if he can't do that, it's time to find another doctor. This stuff they used to do about "protecting" the patient was ridiculous then, and it's even more ridiculous now. Besides, if he's talking to you and not his patient, unless the patient is mentally incompetent or a minor child, he's committing malpractice and you don't want him laying a finger on someone you love anyway!

Still, some doctors do avoid telling their patients bad news. My friend Frank got frustrated by his first doctor, but couldn't figure out what the problem was. I helped him figure out that the doctor wasn't communicating well, so Frank didn't truly understand what was wrong. I would ask simple questions about what the doctor had said, and Frank wouldn't be able to answer; he would complain that the doctor was unclear, or say that they were scheduling him for more tests before they'd tell him anything. The doctor he was with at that time wasn't a specialist and didn't seem to remember Frank's symptoms or have a good grasp of what was wrong with him whenever Frank had an appointment. He even scheduled Frank for a test requiring contrast when Frank had already told him that he had an allergy to contrast! So when I put all of these factors together and showed Frank the pattern, he realized that he needed a different doctor—and he got the "bad news" pretty quickly too, and found that it really wasn't all that bad.

For centuries, physicians often told family members about a patient's medical condition and did not tell the patient, believing it to be too much stress for the patient to handle. Until recently in the United States, patients were specifically not told about a cancer diagnosis because it was equated with an automatic "death sentence." This thinking has changed in recent decades for many reasons.

First of all, cancer is becoming a treatable illness, and there is a greater probability that people with cancer will survive this disease rather than die of the cancer. Second, because of the all the treatment possibilities and side effects of these treatments, patients themselves need to be aware of what they will be going through so that they can make good, informed decisions about what treatments they choose to take. Third, ethically and legally in the United States, patients need to be told about their disease and about all reasonable treatments in a process called **informed consent**. Informed consent is based on the idea that individuals should make decisions for themselves. It is a crucial process of communication between physician and patient (and her family, if she chooses), and often entails patients signing forms indicating their understanding and agreement to certain procedures and treatments.

There are a few exceptions to adult patients providing informed consent. Patients can be deemed **incapacitated** for the purpose of making medical decisions, in which case a **surrogate decision-maker** or **health care proxy** provides consent for procedures or treatments. However, even if a patient is deemed incapacitated and cannot provide informed consent, physicians usually try to give a patient as much information as possible, even if the proxy is the official decision-maker. In other circumstances, a patient may explicitly state to the physician that he or she does not want to know anything about the disease or treatments, designating a person with whom the physician can communicate and obtain informed consent. How this is handled depends on the individual physician and hospital policies. Or, in rare cases, a physician can determine that a clinical exception should be made, indicating that telling the patient about a medical issue would cause

Informed consent

after a patient is educated about his or her diagnosis and all reasonable procedures and treatments options for the disease, he or she must indicate an understanding and agreement to a course of action by signing forms.

Incapacitated

term used when a patient is deemed by the medical team as being unable to give informed consent for a medical procedure (i.e., comatose, mentally disoriented).

Surrogate decision-maker

a person designated to make health-related decisions of that patient. The medical team addresses all health-care issues for the patient directly to the surrogate.

Health care proxy

a document (also called medical durable power of attorney or health care agent) designating a family member, guardian, or friend as the decision-maker about medical treatment for a patient.

so much psychological and emotional harm to a patient that it could affect the medical condition or safety of the patient. For example, a physician may postpone talking about the cancer with a patient with severe depression or with one who is actively suicidal until he or she is psychiatrically stable.

Cultural circumstances may impact whether family members want a patient to be told "bad news," such as the initial cancer diagnosis or the spread of the cancer. In some cultures, it is common for adult children to completely manage their parents' medical care, including speaking with the physicians, deciding about treatment, and so forth. However, in the United States, these cultural standards are sometimes in conflict with the legal standards and ethics in medicine. Communication with the doctor, patient, and family can often clarify such concerns.

Physicians may tell the family more about a patient's illness than they tell the patient. Initially, you may think this is a good idea. However, we have found that it can be difficult for the more informed family members for many reasons, not the least being that they know a "secret" that the patient does not know about her own body. Secrets are often disruptive to communication, since family members have to hold back their emotional reactions to the news to "protect" the patient. This can create distrust between the patient and the family (since patients almost always realize when things are not being told to them) or between the patient and her physician if the patient does not believe the doctor is being truthful with her.

In summary, unless there is a really good reason not to tell your mother, she should be told about the news, no matter what it is, ideally directly from the physician herself. Try not to take on the "go-between" role of relating information from the physician to your mother, since this can be a very stressful role for you to assume. If the physician tells you things in the future, you may want to direct her to your mother and have the discussion together. Patients usually find out the truth anyway, and it is the not knowing that increases their sense of being out of control. We have found that patients usually handle things better than their family and doctors expected, and that information is a crucial part of patients establishing a sense of control. Not knowing, as our patients often say, is worse than knowing the worst.

Patients usually handle things better than their family and doctors expected.

58. I have two children. I don't want to tell them about my wife's diagnosis and surgery because I don't want to upset them. I can barely handle this myself, so how can they cope with the cancer? Should I tell them about the cancer, and if so, how much?

Telling your children about your wife's cancer diagnosis is one of the most difficult issues you may have to face as a parent. Some people are reluctant to tell their children; whereas, others want to be as open as possible. Research and our professional experience as oncology counselors indicate that telling children the truth from the beginning generally leads to better adjustment. However, as their parent, you are the expert on your children, and you should keep them as involved only as much as you and they feel comfortable. Furthermore, as the "well" parent or family member, you may be able to play a valuable role in establishing communication with your children, since oftentimes the parent with cancer is unavailable (in the hospital, for example), and you may spend more time with the children due to increased childcare responsibilities when your spouse is not feeling well.

Obviously, the ages of children affect what type and how much information they can comprehend. For example, a 4-year-old will not understand as much detail as a 10-year-old, nor will a 10-year-old understand as much as a teenager. However, the following guidelines may be helpful and, unless otherwise stated, are good points to keep in mind for all age groups of children. A grandparent (or other family member) may also find the information below helpful.

- Children have a good sense for what is going on with the person with cancer and the family. They often observe subtle changes as well as obvious ones (e.g., concerns about hospital bills or overhearing you or a family member on the phone). Therefore, they may know about the diagnosis anyway, and maybe they should hear it from you or your spouse—the earlier, the better. This is a time to develop trust with your child regarding the diagnosis and treatment.
- Because every type of cancer is different, and each person's treatment is individually tailored, you need to give your children the opportunity to ask about your wife's cancer and treatments so that they do not get misinformation (from the Internet, gossip, family friends, relatives, or other children).

- The word "cancer" is an abstract term that is often hard for children to understand, which can lead to increased fear and misunderstanding. Showing children age-appropriate pictures and diagrams of the body, including where the cancer is located—or especially for younger children, allowing them to draw pictures of it themselves—will help them conceptualize the cancer. One 6-year-old girl drew a picture of her father with a big black dot on his "tummy," representing the cancer. This picture made it much easier for her to visualize and talk about the cancer with her parents.

- Your children may react differently after they discuss the cancer with you and your spouse. Some children, especially very young children, can digest only bits of information at a time. They may not ask questions initially, so make sure that the "big talk" is not just a one-time thing. Continue to check in with your children to see how they are doing and to tell them how you are doing, too. However, if they do not want to talk, do not push them. Instead, explain to them that they can ask you or your wife any questions they like, which gives them control. Remember that if you have more than one child, each one may react differently. Think about whether you want to talk to your children together or individually. One compromise is to have a family meeting first and then follow up with each child separately.

- Children often focus on how cancer will affect their lives, occasionally appearing selfish and expressing anger and frustration. Teenagers and children may resent being asked to help with household duties to help a sick parent. Try to be patient with a child who expresses these feelings and to understand without judgment (which can be difficult). Try to find solutions, such as temporarily hiring a housekeeper or asking family or neighbors to help with household chores so that household routines are less disrupted.

- Providing physical reassurance, such as hugs and touch, is important to you and your children, especially infants or toddlers, for whom modes of communication are limited. Your wife may not be able to play "rough" with your children immediately after surgery or because of fatigue, so explain this to your children and substitute other activities and forms of physical connection (such as sitting closely together, watching a video, or reading together). You do not want them to mistake a lack of physical attention as rejection.

- Continue (as much as possible) with pre-cancer routines and disciplinary actions. This may be difficult because you have demands on your time, but try to allow your child to remain in his or her activities, see friends, and get up in the morning and go to bed at the same times. Some parents want to be more indulgent, and some more strict; however, this is not going to make your child cope any better. Consistency communicates security to children.

Tip: Be honest and consistent, and reassure your child that the cancer is no one's fault.

59. Is it OK to bring a child to the hospital?

Mark's comment:

Children have the right to see their sick grandparent or parent, dying or not. Death is part of life, and though this might be the first time the child sees it, it won't be the last—

so don't treat it like it's some great horror or mystery for the kid to be afraid of. Kids get more upset if they're not allowed to say their goodbyes to dying relatives, so you're not doing them any favors by keeping them out of the sick room.

Some children become very involved and interested in cancer and treatment. They may even want to attend appointments or visit their parent at the hospital. Allowing them to attend an appointment (after first discussing this with your physician and establishing guidelines) may be a good way for them to be reassured and have the opportunity to ask questions. However, it is important not to overwhelm them with information; otherwise, this meeting may make them more anxious and have the opposite effect of what was intended.

Children who want to go to chemotherapy or visit the hospital should be prepared beforehand. Tell them about the treatments and about what they might see (including tubes, other sick patients, and so on). Taking a picture of your wife in treatment can also help them visualize what they might see before they arrive. Some children want to learn about all the tubes, stitches, and other accessories of treatment. Feel free to give them as much information as you, and they, feel comfortable with. Remember, you are the expert on your child, so pay attention to your instincts, and stop when you feel he or she has experienced enough.

Ask about your hospital's policies before bringing your child to visit.

Since most hospitals have visiting hours and policies that may restrict child visitors under a certain age, ask about your hospital's policies before bringing your child to visit.

Relationship and Family Issues

60. Our children haven't said much since their father was diagnosed with cancer, but we've noticed that they're trying almost too hard to help out at home, which is definitely a change. Is this normal?

Children often blame themselves for problems, including a parent's cancer diagnosis. Many children create fantasies to explain events. They might think that their father got cancer because they were not doing well in school or because they shouted something at him or secretly wished that something bad would happen to him the last time they were punished. Because children often think that they did something to cause the cancer, they sometimes think that they have the power to make it go away. A youngster may become the "model child" and try to do everything right. A teenager may suddenly become overly helpful around the house or the play the role of "substitute parent."

Sometimes parents mistake this exemplary behavior to mean that their child is coping well. However, being "perfect" can be a tremendous burden for your child because of the feelings of responsibility that this method of coping entails. Children may fear that if they "mess up," they will make the ill parent worse; if a complication occurs, they may feel guilty that they did not try hard enough to be perfect. You may be surprised at what your children may be thinking. Ask them. They need reassurance that they are neither the cause of the cancer nor responsible for making it go away.

61. What if my child asks: "Is Mommy going to die?"

Children of all ages often ask the "hard" questions that adults have learned not to blurt out. For example, sometimes the first question out of a younger child's mouth after being told a parent has cancer is "Is Mommy (or Daddy) going to die?" This is the hard one. Not only can it bring up tremendous feelings of fear and anxiety in you, but it is also the time when most parents want to reassure their child (and themselves) that everything is going to be OK and that, of course, Mommy (or Daddy) will not die, will never die.

However, this is simply not true. Just as flowers and pets will die, everyone dies at some point. While it is important that you reassure your child, do not misrepresent the truth. You can say something like, "Yes, Mommy does have cancer. However, she is getting the best treatment and seeing the best doctors who are going to try everything to fight this cancer. Everyone dies someday, but we are going to battle this cancer with all our might." If they have known someone else to die from cancer, you need to reassure them that this is not necessarily going to happen to their mother. Give your child age-appropriate specifics about the cancer and treatment, including how Mom's cancer is different from other situations your child may know about (such as a grandmother who died of cancer).

62. How do I know if my children are having problems coping?

Kathleen McCue, the author of *How to Help Children Through a Parent's Serious Illness*, describes some of the warning signs to look out for: major changes or disturbances in sleeping or eating; the appearance of new fears that won't go away; retreating into silence; and trouble with developmental milestones (for example, a potty-trained toddler who starts to wet the bed or a teenager's drop in grades at school). See the Appendix for the full reference to this very helpful book.

If you are unsure about how to talk to your child or have concerns about how he or she is coping with the diagnosis, speak to a social worker or counselor who specializes in helping children of a parent with cancer. If your children are in school, talking with their teachers and/or a school counselor can be helpful, too. Take steps to ensure that significant adults (such as caregivers, close family members, and teachers) around your child are providing consistent messages. You may want to tell these adults generally what your wife is going through medically and what your child already knows. These people will be able to provide support to your child and also notify you if they have concerns about how your child is coping. If you have concerns about how your children are coping with the diagnosis, you can investigate counseling for your children or groups intended specially for children coping with a parent diagnosed with cancer.

63. My friend is a single mother of two young children. Even though she is doing fine medically since her cancer diagnosis, she would like to make plans for the care of the children if something should happen to her. Is this possible? If so, what do I do to help her?

Thousands of children are orphaned every year due to the death of a parent. The care of these children after a parent's death is often not planned for. Subsequently, these children may be placed in foster care, be adopted, or subject to other legal and non-legal arrangements, often causing disruption and trauma to the children involved. To avoid confusion, reduce trauma to the children and potential guardians, and to increase the peace of mind of the parent, a **standby guardian** can be legally designated. A parent, such as your friend who is diagnosed with a life-threatening illness, can identify a standby guardian in case something happens to her in the future—either due to this illness or for another reason.

Securing standby guardianship for children is a very difficult thing for any parent to do. It represents an acknowledgment that it's possible she may not live long enough to see her children grow up, and accepting this reality is the initial, but most difficult step. It sounds as if your friend has already come to this realization. And, even though she is doing well medically now, she is putting her children's needs first by wanting to make plans for their future if something does happen to her.

There are many ways you can help her. Be there to talk to her about her feelings, thoughts, and plans for her

Standby guardian
legally designated person who will have custody of a patient's children in the event of their parent's death or mental incapacitation.

children. If she does not have a specific person or couple in mind as potential guardians, then she may need your support in deciding whom to ask. The first person usually considered is a biological parent (the children's father/s). If this is not possible or recommended, other family members or close friends may be identified. After she has already identified someone, she may need your support talking to that person about her plans. As a friend, you can be there for her for emotional support and guidance.

You may also want to investigate resources for her, such as lawyers who specialize in custody planning. If the patient is not able to afford a lawyer, she can contact agencies to seek assistance, such as the Legal Aid Society or the bar association of the state where she lives. It is important that her plans for guardianship are planned out legally to allow for the smoothest transition, and many resources are available to help her through this process, including the Internet. (See the Appendix for *www.standbyguardianship.org*, a Web site providing state-by-state information regarding standby guardianship legislation, and *www.lawhelp.org*, which is an online legal assistance referral service for people with low to moderate incomes.)

Children should be made aware of the plans for their future.

Children should be made aware of the plans for their future, and they should talk about this with their mother, if possible. As a friend, you can help arrange these discussions between the patient and her children if she is finding it difficult to do so. Children need to know that their mother is taking care of them, no matter what happens. They may be sad and upset, understandably, but the fewer surprises they experience, the better they will cope. If your friend does die from this disease, you can be there to help her children adjust to her death. Knowing of your support now and in the future may be particularly comforting to your friend.

64. My husband is not sure whether he wants to tell anyone about his diagnosis. I believe that I have to let some family members and friends know what's going on. Whom do I tell, what do I tell them, and how will they react?

Some people do not tell anyone anything (sometimes not even their spouses) about the cancer diagnosis, whereas others tell the world everything (literally, by writing books about their experiences). While telling no one can lead to lack of support and isolation, disclosure is a highly personal decision, and one that patients should have as much control over as possible.

Discussions about medical issues and body functions are usually kept private in our society. It's natural for people to be unsure of how much to tell others. After learning about your husband's cancer, such as where in the body it is located and about the functions of that body part, both of you may begin to practice talking about his diagnosis with close, trusted friends and family. See how they react and what questions they ask. Often, knowing what other people think and the questions they ask helps patients and family members prepare themselves for what to tell other people. If you and your husband feel comfortable and choose to tell other people, start talking about his diagnosis more openly. If it fits with your personality, humor is often a good icebreaker and can make you and others feel more at ease. As patients learn more about their cancer, prognosis, and treatment plan—and the helpful role that family and friends can play in this process—they may become more comfortable generally talking about their illness.

Keep in mind that you and your husband may have different ideas regarding who, what, and how to tell others. He may need more time than you do to adjust to the diagnosis, or he may feel that he wants to keep this information confidential. You and your husband may want to specify what you are going to tell other people if they ask you questions, so that you are providing consistent information.

Remember, people you tell will have their own conceptions about cancer. If you decide to disclose the diagnosis, be prepared for a variety of reactions to the news. For some, talking about cancer elicits fear and misunderstanding, and they may want to avoid the topic. Some people wrongly believe that cancer is contagious or that cancer is always terminal. Some patients and family members have felt rejected by others' unintentional reactions, sometimes from close friends who do not call anymore or do not want to socialize. On the other hand, other friends or even distant acquaintances may offer their support. Old friendships can grow and new friendships bloom.

Some people may be very interested in your husband's diagnosis, treatment, and even prognosis. For these reactions, provide only as much information as *he and you* feel comfortable providing—don't feel pressured to divulge too much. People may also want to share their own experiences with cancer or information that they think will be helpful. Some family members have found advice and sharing helpful, particularly in the beginning. However, sometimes this information can be confusing, particularly when the information is irrelevant to your situation or when it is upsetting. If you start to feel overwhelmed, simply tell people that you appreciate their concern but that you feel better discussing the medical concerns solely with the doctor. You may hear of, or know of, other people diagnosed with cancer, maybe even the same type of cancer, who are not faring well medically. Remember, however, that every person is different, every cancer is different, and every person's response to treatment is unique.

Most people will be supportive and sensitive to you and your husband's needs and offer support. Be prepared to accept such offers. Do not be afraid to ask for specific help, such as driving your children to their activities, preparing meals, helping with laundry and cleaning, or just doing something fun together. People with whom you share the diagnosis may be relieved when you ask for specific help as it takes pressure off them to try to figure out how to help. They want to feel useful and be involved. Furthermore, by accepting assistance, you may feel less stressed by having fewer drains on your energy.

65. I heard that my wife's cancer may be genetically related. Do other family members have to be told? Should they be encouraged to be tested for cancer themselves?

The first thing your wife needs to do is to sit down with her doctor to clarify what is meant by "genetically related." This term can mean many different things, and you and your wife need to understand exactly what the doctor means by this statement. If the doctor believes your wife's cancer could indicate an increased risk factor for relatives or your children (or future children), you may consider seeking more information from a **genetic counselor** to discuss what is known about her cancer and its connection with genetics. Based on her family history of cancer, or perhaps through further genetic testing, the counselor will be able to make recommendations regarding screening tests for the cancer, which member(s) of the family should undergo these tests, and when. Since the earlier a cancer is diagnosed, the better the chances for cure, this information can be of life-altering importance to other family members.

Genetic counselor

an expert in genetics, a branch of science focused on the transmission and consequences of biologic inheritance.

However, people at higher risk for cancer may avoid getting these tests based on the very powerful fear of finding out that they have the disease or that they have passed on a genetic predisposition for cancer to their children. Similarly, the person with cancer may fear that telling other family members that they are at a higher risk for cancer will cause their loved ones emotional distress.

Talking about personal fears with your spouse and a member of your medical team can help clarify the underlying beliefs causing your resistance. They also may help provide strategies for good communication. For many families informed about their risk of a cancer diagnosis, the bonds of support and love only strengthen.

Clearly, if there is someone in the family who is already extremely emotionally distressed or psychiatri-

Relationship and Family Issues

cally unstable, caution needs to be exercised in passing this information on to that individual. In any case, anyone contemplating testing should be made aware that there are genetic counselors and trained clinicians to help him or her understand the personal risk for developing cancer and how to cope with the psychological challenges that this knowledge can bring. The Appendix contains information to help with issues related to genetic testing and counseling.

66. Since my spouse's diagnosis, it seems that our family has really changed. We have each risen to the challenge, but how much change is good for our family, and how can we keep things as normal as possible?

Cancer affects the entire family, not merely the patient diagnosed with the disease. All family members will react to the news of the cancer diagnosis in their own ways, and each will cope differently. However, despite being unique people, you are also part of one family, and what you each do will affect the rest of the members. All of you are coping with the normal reactions to the cancer and feeling appropriate emotions; in addition, daily life may be altered. The person diagnosed with cancer may not be able to fulfill his or her household chores or professional obligations due to medical treatment or physical changes, and the role of other family members may need to adjust to compensate. For example, if long-distance family members come to the patient's home to help care for the patient, having another person around, no matter how helpful and loving, is still a change to which your family needs to adapt.

Cancer affects the entire family, not merely the patient.

Keeping family life as normal as possible is a good goal, but be flexible if modifications to your normal routine are needed or unavoidable. For example, try to go to bed and wake up at the same times you are used to, eat meals at the same time, and keep up with physical activity. After the initial crisis of the diagnosis, make a point to socialize, attend religious services, and enjoy other activities. Still clean the house, do the laundry and other chores (as much as possible). Not only is maintaining a daily routine practical (the dishes will be done!), but it is also comforting to keep things consistent at a time when uncertainty about medical issues is high. Children, in particular, respond well to keeping a normal routine. Furthermore, doing things not related to the diagnosis can be a practical temporary distraction from the doctors, the hospital, and other reminders of the cancer.

Hopefully, a "new normal" for your family will be established with time. As you begin to understand more about the disease, its symptoms, and your loved one begins treatments, these aspects of the cancer will become part of your "new normal." Talk with your family members, including your spouse, about what the change has been like for them. Communication not only can allow people to vent their feelings, but it can also be an effective way for you to identify tensions and find solutions to ensure that life proceeds as normally as possible. If you believe that your family needs help communicating or adjusting to the diagnosis, family therapy can be helpful. You may want to contact your hospital social worker or investigate local family therapists.

Maintaining normal routines does not mean that you should be inflexible if alterations in your life need to be made. It also does not mean that the family needs to "pretend" that everything is wonderful. Try to strike a balance between maintaining consistency, but be willing to change, since sticking to harsh regimens can exacerbate tensions.

67. Like any family, we have members who don't get along, complicated by long-term, unresolved problems, divorces, etc. Is there any way to minimize these tensions, at least while we are dealing with this cancer?

Mark's comment:

The only thing you can really do is talk honestly with all the people involved. If they're not willing to put aside their problems, at the very least, ask them not to aggravate the situation by airing grievances in these circumstances. If they must have a fight, they can have it somewhere other than in front of the person who's sick.

The emotional impact of the diagnosis sometimes brings family members together in positive ways, even those who previously did not get along well. Family members express their hope that they can all put aside their personal differences and come together to support the patient, and each other, during the cancer crisis. Often, this way of coping is ideal and is the hope of patients who feel they have enough to worry about with the cancer and do not want to have this crisis complicated by family disagreements.

However, sometimes family members cannot put the past behind them, and the family problems they had before the diagnosis may continue or even increase during the diagnosis and treatment. The stress of cancer and treatments may worsen already strained relationships. Modern families are also complicated by divorces, remarriages, step-family members, and so forth, and family roles can be confused. For example, an adult child may feel that he should be the primary caregiver and decision-maker rather than a new spouse by remarriage.

Such tensions can be hard to resolve and may be impossible to avoid. Open communication about each person's beliefs and feelings can sometimes reduce tensions. A truce, of sorts, can often be arranged while important medical decisions need to be made and/or the patient would benefit from a united family support system.

Tensions may also arise if you think that others are not doing enough or not providing needed support. It is sometimes helpful to designate a "coordinator" of care. Think about designating someone in the family who is least caught up in the tensions and whom other family members will most likely follow. This person can arrange schedules for the rest of the family, including providing transportation to and from appointments, preparing meals, cleaning the house, going grocery shopping, and helping the patient do activities such as getting a haircut, attending church/religious services, going shopping or to sports events. The patient may also serve in this role of care organizer, if he or she wants to. Family members who are willing and able to be involved can be included in caregiving responsibilities, if this is what the patient wishes. For example, a spouse may not be able to attend all medical appointments with the patient. Perhaps other family members can share in this responsibility by taking turns driving and providing support to the patient. Allow the patient to identify his or her needs, and then start to assign tasks. This way everyone will feel he or she is contributing.

Disagreement about medical decisions is another common source of tension among family members. Family members may disagree with who should do what, when, and how. Every person, even if he or she grew up in the same family, brings different perspectives and values to making important decisions. The patient may seek family input if a decision needs to be made, such as starting, changing, or stopping treatment for the cancer. Emotions run high during such times. However, keep in mind that the patient is the one making the decisions. If he or she seeks out one or two people with whom to consult, honor this decision. If the patient makes choices you personally do not agree with, you may want to discuss this, calmly, but always remember that medical decisions are up to the patient, not you or other family members. Supporting decisions that the patient makes is an important, yet sometimes difficult job for the family.

Remember that medical decisions are up to the patient, not you or other family members.

If the patient becomes unable to make decisions on her behalf, a surrogate or health care proxy should have been previously identified by the patient. This person has the legal right to make decisions on behalf of the patient. However, this does not mean that close family members should not be involved in the decisions. Hopefully, the patient has identified a surrogate/health care proxy and discussed her wishes in advance, reducing possible tensions among family members. Seeking out health care professionals to help coordinate the decision-making process often helps reduce frustration and conflict. Refer to Question 94 to learn more about health care proxies and surrogate decision-making.

Keep in mind that your perceptions of a family member's reactions are colored by your past experiences with that person. Try to start with a clean slate when dealing with the diagnosis and subsequent family input. Put the past aside as much as possible and realize that each family member will react to the diagnosis and the added responsibilities in different ways. Some people may use denial and/or avoidance as their method of coping—they simply may not be able to handle the emotions as well as others. Speaking to such a person compassionately may help him or her feel better—maybe he or she can become more involved by doing fun activities with the patient, instead of staying for long visits at the hospital or attending medical appointments—both of which may be overwhelming.

Realize, however, that no matter how hard you try, you may not be able to resolve tensions in the family or change others' reactions or behaviors. Focus on what you can do to help the patient, your family, and yourself. If you pay more attention to yourself and your own reactions to stress, and think less about other people's reactions, they may bother you less often. Additionally, tensions may ease if family members set an example of putting the past behind them and focusing on the present situation.

68. My partner and I are in a committed relationship, but are not married. How will this affect us?

Non-married partners may face added challenges when one person is diagnosed with cancer. These challenges can be broken down into several categories: interpersonal, legal, and financial.

First, define your relationship to yourself and ask yourself practical questions, such as: How involved are you going to be in your partner's medical care and decisions? Have you spoken to her about her wishes on these matters? Are you going to be a primary contact for the doctors and nurses, or is someone else in her family? Are you going to be able to provide personal care to your loved one if she becomes too debilitated to care for herself (temporarily or permanently)? Think about these important issues, and then discuss them with your partner. A cancer diagnosis can make both people think about the level of commitment in their relationship and hopefully discuss these issues openly.

Partners of patients, whether they are in a heterosexual or same-sex relationship, may sometimes feel ignored in the medical setting or marginalized by the patient's family members. If you feel that you are being overlooked by the medical staff, or by other involved family members, speak with the patient first, if possible. If you and your partner agree that you are the primary caregiver and/or should be privy to medical information, your partner should make this clear to her doctors and family.

At many hospitals visitors are restricted to spouses and "family members," particularly in critical situations, and hospitals may not provide medical information over the telephone. Family members not supportive of your relationship may try to exclude you from discussions with the doctor, decision-making, and even prevent you from visiting the patient. Protect yourself and the patient by establishing your relationship and involvement with medical decisions from the very beginning. **Patient confidentiality** concerns limit what medical professionals can tell people other than

Patient confidentiality

legal limits as to what the medical team can tell people other than the patient and his or her spouse or designated surrogate/health care proxy.

121

the patient about the patient's medical care. If your loved one agrees, she or he should ask the doctor to clearly indicate in the medical record that you are able to receive information about the patient's condition or medical details in person or via telephone and have visiting privileges. Additionally, you should always carry a copy of the signed health care proxy if you are identified as the surrogate.

Same-sex couples sometimes face discrimination by medical professionals. In addition to the financial and legal protections mentioned in this book, you may also want to talk with a community agency specializing in gay/lesbian/transgender concerns. Advocates there may have additional suggestions on how to protect yourselves legally (since this can vary from state to state), financially, and emotionally.

Both married and non-married couples need to budget for unexpected costs related to the cancer diagnosis, such as transportation, insurance premiums and co-pays, and reduced income if the patient is unable to work. Whether or not you and your partner keep your finances separate, the two of you should discuss the level of financial responsibility you are able, and will-ing, to contribute. Financial issues are among the most stressful issues with which couples coping with cancer grapple, and more planning can reduce tension in your relationship.

You want to be sure that your stake in any common property or combined finances is legally recognized. For example, domestic partners sometimes have their home in just one person's name, even though both contribute to the house payments. If something should happen to either one of you, your investment in this property may not be recognized if your name is not on the title or lease. In other words, you may lose money and property if you are not legally protected. Each state has unique laws pertaining to non-married partners, and you should speak with a lawyer to discuss ways to protect yourselves. For example, property may need to be in both of your names, and each of you should have a **last will and testament**. You may also want to discuss other financial issues with an accountant or financial planner. Some people choose to put finances in a **living trust**, transfer funds into the well partner's account, establish financial **power of attorney**, or open joint banking accounts so that finances are less likely to be contested by other people.

There are other non-financial legal considerations that you may discuss with a lawyer. If you serve as your partner's primary caregiver and/or he wants you to serve as his health care surrogate decision maker, you should make sure that he has identified you as such in writing—in some states this is called a health care proxy form. He may also see a lawyer to give you his power of attorney regarding his health care. If your partner does *not* specify you as the surrogate decision maker, you may not have this right. In fact, in most states, family members may have the legal right to perform this role, thus potentially excluding you from any involvement. You may also want to make sure that relevant family members know that you are identified as the surrogate and what your partner's wishes are. This may prevent crises and tensions between his family members and you, particularly if your partner is ever mentally incapacitated and medical decisions need to be made.

Relationship and Family Issues

Last will and testament

legal document specifying a person's wishes with regards to inheritance after the person dies.

Living trust

a legal document created for a person while he or she is still alive in order to protect financial assets. A financial planner or lawyer can provide details.

Power of Attorney

a surrogate or proxy decision maker for the patient who legally makes all health-related and financial decisions for the patient; entails a legal document.

69. Now that my wife has completed cancer treatment, how do we move forward with our lives?

Advances in the early diagnosis and treatment of cancer are increasing the number of people who survive the disease. This also means that there is an increasing number of patients and families who need input about putting their cancer behind them and moving forward again. This may seem an easy adjustment to some people, but for others, it is not. They may ask themselves, "Isn't this what I have dreamed about since the diagnosis? Shouldn't we be grateful she survived the cancer?" However, the following issues may arise for both patients and family members during the post-treatment phase and complicate the process of cancer recovery:

- Fear of cancer recurrence
- Changed self-esteem and self-image
- Legal and financial issues after diagnosis (e.g., initiating a new job search, writing "the right résumé," etc.)
- Concern about possible genetic predisposition of cancer in family members
- Concern about future medical issues, follow-up, and screening
- Leading a healthy lifestyle, including exercising, stopping smoking, changing dietary habits
- Unresolved life issues that were postponed because of diagnosis and treatment (such as marrying or separating, having children, or changing careers)
- Long-term treatment side effects, such as scars, ostomy, infertility, and sexual issues

Often, techniques used for coping with cancer diagnosis and treatment help patients and their spouses develop a broader understanding of life that includes all of their experiences, including surviving cancer. However, sometimes after treatment, survivors and their families experience new problems in coping and need to investigate new avenues to help themselves. For some who coped well during the whole diagnosis and treatment phase, the realization of the cancer experience sometimes hits them long after the ordeal is over. If you or your wife experience some problems moving forward, you may want to find a support group, another survivor, or an oncology mental health professional to help you understand and manage these issues as you work toward restoring your quality of life. Further information is available at survivorship programs at many cancer centers, such as the Post Treatment Resource Program at Memorial Sloan-Kettering Cancer Center, as well as the American Cancer Society and Cancer Care, Inc. (See the Appendix for further information).

PART SIX

Home Care, Medical Equipment, Place- ment, and Other Practical Matters

What is home care? What can we expect from home care after surgery and during other treatments?

What is a skilled nursing facility? How do you get in?

The doctors want my husband to get radiation ther- apy for the next six weeks, five days a week. I don't drive, and I'm afraid my husband won't feel well enough after his treatments to drive himself. How is he going to get back and forth from his treatments?

More ...

70. *What is home care? What can we expect from home care after surgery and during other treatments?*

Home care is a broad term used to describe many types of medical and/or personal care services provided in a person's home. Multiple terms used for different types of care are often confusing, so be specific about your wants and needs when you discuss home care options. Medical home care often requires a doctor's order and usually involves **skilled nursing needs** such as open wound care, checks of vital signs, or infusion care.

A **home health aide** (sometimes also referred to as a personal care attendant) is a person who is qualified to provide "personal care," such as assisting someone with bathing, dressing, and getting around. They most often work for a home health care agency and may also assist with light housework. A home health aide is not usually covered by insurance unless it is ordered in conjunction with a skilled nursing need. A home attendant (or homemaker care) is a person who can assist with shopping, house cleaning, doing laundry, cooking, and accompanying a person to appointments, and whose services are usually not covered by most insurance policies.

A common misperception among patients and family is that they will automatically have insurance-covered home care provided after their discharge from an inpatient hospital admission, particularly after surgery. Most insurance companies cover only skilled nursing needs, usually requiring a registered nurse, a physical therapist, an occupational therapist, or someone with other medical expertise. In addition to covering these

---

Home care

medical, nursing, social, or rehabilitative services provided in the patient's home.

Skilled nursing need

a need for services or care that can be performed only by a licensed nurse, such as treating a wound, teaching the administration of new medications, or assessing the clinical status at home. Often a requirement for home care by insurers.

Home health aide

qualified person able to assist a patient with bathing, dressing, getting around in his or her own home, and doing other homemaking tasks.

skilled medical needs, policies sometimes cover a limited number of home health aide hours (most often fewer than 20 hours a week, if at all).

Patients and family may feel cheated if they were expecting more professional assistance to be covered by insurance. This is an upsetting situation that can be avoided with advance preparation. Contact the insurance carrier for your loved one and ask about home care coverage and what, exactly, is needed for coverage (for example, physician certification of a skilled nursing need). Furthermore, it is important for patients and family members to understand the limits of home care and begin to make arrangements early for caring for the patient at home. This may entail family members helping the recuperating patient after discharge with cooking, cleaning and other needs, and/or providing other types of assistance, such as transportation to follow-up doctor visits. Family members may also need to learn to do wound dressing changes, take care of drains or other medical home equipment or needs.

If home care is ordered by the doctor and covered by a patient's insurance, the discharge planning staff member (often a social worker or nurse case manager) will discuss the type of care the patient will receive and when the initial home visit will take place. Sometimes the home care agency will contact you directly to establish the details after the formal referral has been made by the discharge planning staff. Often a first visit from an intake registered nurse will take place one day to several days after discharge. The nurse will assess the patient's needs and the home environment to determine the type of care, the frequency of visits, and any equipment/supply needs that may be required. Be sure to accurately describe your loved one's diagnosis, surgery, or other treatment side effects as well as any other concerns or questions you have about managing at home.

Before your loved one leaves the hospital, be sure to get the names and numbers of the discharge planner (or whoever you should contact at the hospital if you have problems with the home care that is ordered), the name of the home care agency, and whom you should contact in case of a medical emergency (even after business hours). This information should be located on discharge papers you receive the day of discharge from the hospital. Patients and family sometimes leave the hospital without these crucial contact numbers, which can cause added stress if they have a question later. If this information is not given to you, or if you misplace it, ask for it and keep it handy so that you can refer to it when needed.

In addition to medical home care and family or friend caregivers, you might also want to investigate community agencies that provide various services to a person's home, such as Meals on Wheels (where low-cost, prepared meals are delivered directly to your home); senior centers; private nonprofit organizations that serve senior citizens or disabled individuals; volunteer agencies; and churches, synagogues, and other religious centers. Furthermore, there are long-term care policies and supplemental insurance coverage may be available to purchase even after the cancer diagnosis. Contact your state's insurance department for a list of companies that sell long-term care insurance or check with your current medical insurance provider for purchasing additional coverage.

If you feel that you and your loved one cannot manage safely or easily at home, discuss other options with your family and discharge planner. These can include private pay home care, nursing home placement, or assisted living options. NewLifeStyles (see the Appendix) is a good resource for investigating the types of home care, facility placement, and other alternative living arrangements (such as "assisted living"). We discuss facility placement options in Question 74.

71. My husband just had colon surgery, and we were just told by the doctor that he no longer needs to stay in the hospital. Are we really going to be able to manage his care at home?

Nancy's comment:

A visiting nurse can show the caregiver and family simple nursing skills that they can use when home health care persons aren't present. These include using a draw sheet to move a patient in bed, how to pick up someone who has fallen, helping the patient with a bed bath, or how to give a massage. It's important to know how to do these things properly, particularly if you're caring for an elderly person or someone who is physically frail.

In recent years, hospital admissions have gotten shorter, in part because patients can now be sent home to manage their care themselves. With training and reinforcement from inpatient staff and/or visiting nurses, patients and their family caregivers can learn to do injections, manage the intravenous infusion of fluids, and operate feeding tubes or drains on their own.

Sometimes this is for a short time, until the problem resolves and the patient no longer requires the treatment or care. Sometimes, when there are permanent physical changes, as in the creation of a colostomy that diverts solid waste through a surgically created opening in the abdomen, the care regimen can be permanent.

Take steps right from the beginning to prevent yourself from becoming overwhelmed. For example, meet with the nurses and physicians in charge of your husband's care as soon as possible during his hospitalization and establish realistic goals. Keep in mind that your husband's psychological and physical adjustment to surgery—and your adjustment as a caregiving partner—are not going to occur overnight. Pace yourself. If your husband has the medical need, he will most likely have a home care nurse visit and possibly other care services, after he is discharged from the hospital to provide additional instruction and support. Furthermore, community support groups such as the American Cancer Society (ACS) and other agencies can help you and your spouse adjust to body changes after surgery and other treatments.

It's not uncommon for patients and family caregivers to be anxious prior to discharge from the hospital. They are losing the emotional safety net of round-the-clock care from doctors and nurses. Going home and assuming responsibility for your loved one's care will be less intimidating if you focus on getting answers to the following questions before you leave the hospital. If a nurse's visit at home has been arranged, it pays to go over the following questions with the nurse again:

- What can I expect at home?
- What will I have to do?

- What are the potential problems that could arise? What are the warning signs?
- When should I seek professional help, and whom do I call?

These questions are based on a problem-solving approach advocated by American Cancer Society in one of their publications, *Caregiving: A Step-by-Step Resource for Caring for the Person with Cancer at Home* (2000). This book, which we highly recommend, also has numerous chapters devoted to physical conditions (such as pain, fever, and diarrhea) that might occur at home and how to manage them.

72. Can we get a hospital bed for my husband when he returns home from the hospital?

Durable medical equipment (sometimes referred to as "DME"), such as walkers, wheelchairs, bedside commodes, or hospital beds, can be obtained for long-term or short-term use from equipment suppliers. Medical equipment can be delivered to patients' homes while they are still in the hospital or after they are discharged. Check first with the medical team, however, to make sure they agree that the equipment is necessary and appropriate. You will need a doctor's certification of the medical need for the equipment in order to get approval from the insurance company (assuming, of course, that your policy covers durable medical equipment in the first place) or to authorize payment to the equipment company through Medicare or Medicaid. Although there may be other paperwork, usually what's required is a written prescription from the doctor for equipment, much the same as for prescription

Durable medical equipment (DME)

equipment such as walkers, wheelchairs, bedside commodes, or hospital beds that can be ordered from equipment suppliers for home use.

133

drugs. The next step in the process is to have the discharge planner in the hospital (the social worker or nurse case manager) forward the prescriptions to an equipment supply company, who will then make arrangements with you for delivery. If there are items you desire but are not covered, you can always buy or rent them yourself.

Patients who have already been discharged home, and afterwards find that they need equipment to help facilitate their care, can contact their home care company if they are currently receiving nursing visits. They may be able to have the equipment delivered to the patient's home. Or, you should contact the doctor's office. The physician can provide you with a prescription if the patient needs the equipment for medical reasons. You can then take this prescription to an equipment supply company.

73. My mother can barely get out of bed to go to the bathroom. Even though we've hired an aide to help her at home during part of the day, I'm really concerned about her safety when she's alone. What should we do?

Nancy's comment:

If you're caring for someone who doesn't live with you, it can be helpful to have an occupational therapist (OT) make a home visit to the patient's house to evaluate the patient's needs for safety and mobility. This may be covered by insurance. An OT can suggest placement of grab bars in a bathroom, a ramp rather than steps for easier access, and other safety and comfort measures, which can make a great difference in how the person you're caring for can manage when he or she is alone. Just improving a person's mobility can buoy his or her spirits and speed recovery from a difficult round of chemotherapy or radiation treatment.

There are times when people are unable to manage alone, either because of physical limitations, mental impairment, or both. Decisions about how to handle this involve both practical and emotional considerations. Ask yourself: Is the impairment temporary or treatable? Or is the impairment long-term and not likely to improve? If your mother has recently been in the hospital for a couple of weeks or longer, it may not necessarily be the cancer that leaves her unable to care for herself, but rather the weakening and deconditioning of the body that occurs when people are inactive for prolonged periods of time.

In either case, talk with the doctor to see what she thinks is contributing to your mother's physical condition. Ask her about having a physical therapy evaluation. A physical therapist and **physiatrist** (a doctor who specializes in rehabilitation medicine) will both assess your mother's ability to manage safely at home and suggest a program for her rehabilitation. Similarly, if your mother just had surgery and seems confused or "just not herself," it could be a temporary side effect of the anesthesia or other medications. If this continues, do not be surprised if the physician wishes to consult with doctors from other specialties to discuss possible solutions.

Physiatrist
a doctor who specializes in rehabilitation medicine.

If your mother is currently admitted, it may be that after a few days of physical therapy in the hospital, your mother will be able to return home directly and be able to manage with support from family members staying with her. A physical therapist may be able to visit her at home to help her get back her strength, and a home health aide may be included in these services to help your mother get back on her feet again. With this added assessment and assistance at home to what you've already arranged, your mother may be able to manage well out of the hospital.

Although you may still be uncomfortable with the idea of your mother going home, it's important that you take into account how *she* perceives her care needs, before imposing any plans or solutions. If she feels she can manage at home with the help of an aide, or even by herself, you can voice your concerns and discuss with her additional ways of ensuring her comfort and safety: having more family involved; hiring additional help privately; or installing a **Personal Emergency Response System** (PERS), which she can wear on her person so that she can call for immediate help in a crisis.

Personal Emergency Response System (PERS)

device a patient can wear that can alert emergency help.

On the other hand, it may be that your mother does require a longer or more intensive program of physical therapy to get better, or simply needs more help than can be provided at home. In this case, your mother can transfer from the hospital to a skilled nursing facility for rehabilitation (see description in next question), where she can receive both nursing and personal care around the clock, in addition to participating in a daily program of physical therapy.

Skilled nursing facility (SNF)

a healthcare facility providing short-term nursing care with the aim of having the patient return home or to a family member's home.

74. What is a skilled nursing facility? How does my father get into one?

Skilled nursing facilities (or SNFs) are often confused with nursing homes, both by patients and their families. SNFs provide a higher level of shorter-term care that aims at having patients return home or to a family member's home. Nursing homes, on the other hand, provide primarily long-term, custodial care for patients who can no longer live elsewhere on their own. Although many SNFs began as nursing homes, or have units in them that provide long-term care, they also house rehabilitation units where patients can stay temporarily to receive physical and occupational therapy, until they have regained a level of functioning that allows them to go home. Unlike nursing homes, short-term rehabilitation in an SNF is a stepping stone, a structured setting of care to help patients go home.

Once you've begun the process of considering having your father go to an SNF for short-term rehabilitation, the hospital discharge planner should be able to provide you and your father with a list of local facilities. The discharge planner at the hospital will probably have brochures or even videos on hand to provide you with some background about these places. If you or your father is interested about the type of care provided at an SNF, you can contact the admission office of any facility you are considering and arrange a tour.

Your father doesn't necessarily have to go to an SNF in the town where he lives. If it's more convenient, he can go to a facility closer to you in order to make it easier for you or other family members to visit him, provided there aren't any restrictions based upon his insurance. If you know of any facilities from previous experience or have friends who can make recommendations about places, so much the better. Try to identify about five facilities as potential placements for your father, as your first choice may be full or won't accept your father because they can't meet his medical needs. Consult with the hospital discharge planner so that he or she can put in the necessary paperwork for application to these facilities.

If your father participates in a managed care plan, remember that these care facilities may have to be in-network to be covered by insurance. Most SNFs accept Medicare, but Medicare will cover only the first 20 days of a stay at an SNF fully. After that, there is a co-payment for the next 100 days, after which patients are financially responsible for the costs of their stay. For this reason, some facilities require some kind of finan-cial review as part of the application, in case the patient stays at the SNF longer than anticipated.

Once your father is medically cleared and ready for transfer to an SNF, hopefully you will have already vis-ited your five choices and decided upon your prefer-ences. Sometimes, though, your first choice for placement does not have a bed available, even though they've medically accepted the patient. If you're com-fortable going with a second choice facility that does have a bed ready, fine; keep in mind also that it's always possible to transfer later to another facility if the care provided is not adequate. If there are facilities willing and able to accept your father, but you or your father insists on one in particular, the insurer may inform you that it will no longer pay for his current hospitalization while waiting for a bed at your first choice SNF. Things don't often reach this impasse as long as you've been working in conjunction with the medical team and discharge planner and have made a good faith effort to look at options and consider alternatives.

Another obstacle that can arise is when the SNFs refuse to accept a patient on medical grounds, either because the patient is too high-functioning to require rehabilitation in a facility or has other nursing care needs that the facility is unable to provide. In the latter case, you need to go back to the discharge planner to find other facilities capable of providing the specialized care your father needs. If, on the other hand, your father is now getting out of bed independently, walking without assistance, and meeting other goals, SNF placement may, in fact, not be needed, and going home may be the appropriate plan.

75. The doctors want my husband to get radiation therapy for the next six weeks, five days a week. I don't drive, and I'm afraid my husband won't feel well enough after his treatments to drive himself. How is he going to get back and forth from his treatments?

Insurance policies seldom cover the cost of transportation to and from routine medical appointments, but check his insurance plan anyway, just to be sure. If your husband is being treated at a major cancer center at some distance from where you live, you can ask the doctors at the center if there are other medical centers closer to your home where your husband can receive the same treatments. This will make arranging a transportation schedule easier with the assistance of family and friends who might be able to provide rides for your husband to his appointments.

Sometimes help from friends and family is not enough; you may need to explore other options. One is to pay privately for car service or an **ambulette**, if

Ambulette

transport service for patients, usually a van that can accommodate patients in wheelchairs.

you have the financial resources. Hospitals close to home *may* provide free or low-cost transport services to and from medical treatments, such as radiation therapy or chemotherapy. Financial assistance is also sometimes available from local chapters of national cancer support organizations, such as Cancer Care, Inc. and the American Cancer Society, if you can demonstrate financial need.

Another option is to look into public and non-profit transportation programs for the disabled or aged, if your husband qualifies. Most communities, for example, have **paratransit programs** to complement the local public transportation system. If you are unable to use public transportation because of a physical impairment or medical condition, paratransit may be available to take you door-to-door to your desired destination, for the same cost as taking a bus. Advance reservations are required, however; contact your state or local Department of Transportation for details about their program and how to apply for service. Similarly, there may be van service available for senior citizens in your community, sponsored by the government or by community organizations such as churches and voluntary charities, to help you get back and forth between home and the hospital or clinic.

Paratransit programs

local public transport system for those with a physical impairment or medical condition.

Another problem that can arise, even when patients or family are able to drive, is the availability and cost of parking. A handicapped parking permit, available through your local municipality, may help. You don't need to be wheelchair bound to qualify, but usually a letter from a physician is required. The cost of parking in a parking garage per visit can also quickly add up over time, so if you and your husband are on a fixed income with limited resources, ask the social worker at the hospital or clinic where you are being treated whether there are any philanthropic programs or parking vouchers available either through their institution or organizations like Cancer Care, Inc. that might be able to provide financial assistance.

PART SEVEN

Insurance Issues

How can we protect our family financially while being faced with expensive treatments for cancer?

What if the patient does not qualify for Medicaid?

Prescription drug coverage is getting so expensive, even though we have insurance. Is there anything I can do to reduce this expense?

More ...

76. *How can we protect our family financially while being faced with expensive treatments for cancer?*

Mark's comment:

First of all, you'll need to take a serious look at your finances. If you're self-employed as I was when my mother was sick, find a lawyer and discuss options, such as forming a corporation to limit personal financial liability. Figure out as many tax shelters as possible. Think about limiting the number of business associates you tell about your loved one's cancer— potential clients or partners may assume that you're going to be too busy helping the person with cancer to take on work, and then your business will decline just when you need the income most.

Then… just be a grownup about it, which is harder than it sounds if you're caring for someone. Yes, a certain amount of emotional turmoil is to be expected, but the point is that you and your loved one can't allow the cancer to rule your life. You still have to earn money, you still have to live your life, and the dishes don't wash themselves.

One of the primary causes of stress among people with cancer and their families is coping with the possible financial issues. Financial concerns primarily stem from two sources: 1) the cost of medical care and level of insurance coverage, and 2) the loss of wages caused by temporary or permanent job loss. There are several ways to help reduce the financial impact, including knowing what the person with cancer can do to protect him or herself and knowing about possible government and private financial assistance (see Questions 77–80 and 83).

However, this topic is complex and varies by geographic region and by individual concerns and situations. Consult a social worker, along with a lawyer or financial planner, to obtain specific information. The information below serves as a guide to help you ask the right questions.

77. What is Medicare?

Medicare (United States Social Security Administration) is a federally run health insurance program for people who are either age 65 and over, on **Social Security Disability** (SSD) (see below) for two years, legally blind, or on renal dialysis. The information provided below is a brief outline of the different types of Medicare coverage; for more information refer to official Medicare Web site, *http://www.medicare.gov*.

- Part A: Free to eligible people (paid for by the **Social Security** program), but may be purchased if you have not accrued enough Social Security credits based on your work contribution history. It may cover inpatient hospitalization, skilled nursing facility (with specific limitations), **hospice care**, in-home nursing care, and home health care. Deductibles and co-payments may be required.
- Part B: Purchased by paying monthly premiums. Covers most medical services, lab tests, outpatient hospital services, medical equipment and supplies, and chemotherapy, if administered by your health care provider. If an individual meets **Medicaid** requirements (see Question 78), the premium may be paid as part of a program called Qualified Medicare Beneficiary Program. Medicare typically does not cover prescriptions (those not administered by hospital staff), syringes or insulin for diabetics, experimental treatments, routine medical transporta-

Social Security Disability (SSD)
federally run program that provides a monthly income to disabled workers and their families.

Social Security
federally run program that provides monthly payments to persons over age 65 and family survivors; the amount is calculated from the person's work history.

Hospice care
facility or home care program designed to help the physical and emotional needs of the terminally ill.

Medicaid
federal- and state-funded health insurance program for those on a limited income.

tion (ambulance is covered in specific circumstances), or non-medical or extensive home care services.

- Medicare Supplemental (or "MediGap" Plans): Purchased separately, it is intended to provide additional coverage to people with Medicare, such as prescription drug coverage and other benefits. The government has standardized these plans, and they provide a range of additional coverage. To learn more about these policies, order a copy of the *Guide to Health Insurance for People with Medicare* (U.S. Department of Health and Human Services; see the Appendix for ordering information).

- Medicare Managed Care (Medicare HMOs): Medicare establishes an agreement with certain Medicare HMOs to manage the patient's insurance coverage. The person continues to pay for "Part B." If enrolled in such a program, a person may receive added benefits, such as prescription coverage, coverage for checkups, and preventive health care. He or she will probably be required to choose a primary care physician, and may also have added restrictions, such as being limited to in-network medical care (i.e., can choose only doctors/hospitals from a specific list), be required to pay additional fees, and more.

78. What is Medicaid?

Supplemental Security Income (SSI)

federally run program that provides income to eligible people over age 65, legally blind or disabled, who have a low income, few assets or a limited formal work history.

Medicaid (State Department of Social Services; *http://cms.hhs.gov/medicaid*) is a medical insurance program for people who live on a limited income. Eligibility and coverage differ from state to state, and some states are more restrictive than others about income limits. People may be eligible if they have a low income, have high medical bills, receive **Supplemental Security Income** (SSI), and/or meet specific other requirements, such as citizenship status. Some hospitals can apply for Medicaid while a patient is hospitalized; speak to your hospital's financial services department or social worker to find out more about this potential option. Or, you may contact your local Medicaid office or Social Services department directly; a directory of state programs is located on the Internet.

Medicaid Managed Care is similar to Medicare Managed Care in that some states have allowed Medicaid recipients to enroll in managed care plans. In some states, recipients were automatically enrolled in such programs. However, a person diagnosed with cancer may be able to disenroll from these programs if he or she finds that the managed care policies are too restrictive to obtain appropriate medical care. Contact your managed care insurance carrier or Medicaid office to investigate the disenrollment process.

79. What if the patient does not qualify for Medicaid?

Nonprofit agencies and other community resources can sometimes provide limited, temporary assistance for housing, transportation, and other medical expenses not covered by insurance to qualified individuals. Patients may be required to complete a financial evaluation. Such agencies include Cancer Care, Inc., American Cancer Society, local charities, the Department of Veterans Affairs for qualified veterans, and your hospital's social work department or financial services department (see the Appendix for contact information). However, resources are limited and the availability of funds can change, so contacting these places directly for information is a good idea. It may be necessary for family members to pitch in financially as well.

Sometimes patients have no other option but to utilize their own financial resources, including tapping into savings, selling property, or converting investments into cash. Some IRAs (Individual Retirement Accounts) also have emergency clauses whereby the member can make early withdrawals of money in hardship situations. Members can also borrow from their own contributions at low interest rates before they reach retirement age. Be sure to understand the penalties for early withdrawals.

80. Prescription drug coverage is getting so expensive, even though we have insurance. Is there anything I can do to reduce this expense?

Some pharmaceutical companies provide limited free or reduced-cost prescriptions to qualified individuals as part of "compassionate drug" or "patient assistance" programs. If you are having trouble paying for certain prescriptions, ask your doctor or pharmacist what company makes the drug. Then, contact the company to determine whether it has such a program and how you can apply. You can also try NeedyMeds, Inc. (see the Appendix for Web site information) to find information on specific drug or company programs.

Investigate purchasing supplemental insurance coverage to defray the costs of prescriptions. These plans may be expensive, but could be less than buying pricey drugs. Many states also have pharmaceutical assistance programs that provide financial assistance to defray the costs of medications for the elderly or disabled. Contact Cancer Care, Inc. for a list of states with such programs. You should also contact the office administering the program in your state to make sure your loved one qualifies.

81. What are some tips on negotiating with my partner's insurance company?

As family or a friend of a person with cancer, one of the most helpful things you can do is assist the patient with negotiating with insurance coverage. If the patient wants your involvement, she may have to contact the insurance company, her employer and medical provider to give written permission for you to able to give and receive confidential information. As many of our patients and family members tell us, dealing with the insurance claims can be one of the most stressful aspects of managing cancer treatment.

Contact the health insurance carrier, and if your partner receives insurance benefits through her employer, contact her human resources department to discuss her policy coverage as soon as possible. Many insurance companies have established agreements with certain physicians and hospitals, often called the "in-network" medical providers. Furthermore, in order to access this "network" of medical care, a person may first need to be referred by his or her primary care physician to see a specialist. This type of insurance coverage is sometimes referred to as a managed care plan. Different types of insurance plans exist (such as HMOs, POSs, PPOs, etc.), so be sure to contact the insurance provider to get clarification of what is covered, and what isn't, under the plan. Write down the name of the customer service agent to whom you speak.

Even with the most restrictive managed care plans, however, it still may be possible to receive certain types of cancer treatment out-of-network (from hospitals or doctors who do not have specific agreements with your insurance company), particularly if the treatment is not available by an in-network provider. Be aware that going out-of-network can potentially be more costly if the patient has to pay an "out-of-pocket" share herself. Make sure that you both are fully informed about the coverage policy of the institution where your loved one decides to get treatment. Some insurance carriers assign a caseworker if a patient wants to receive treatment out-of-network (or out-of-state), and this person can be a good resource for any insurance-related questions. Be informed about restrictions, such as in-network and out-of-network paperwork, necessary referrals, and/or pre-certifications. *Make sure that all insurance premiums are paid on time.* Being late or missing a payment can be reason for an insurance company to discontinue coverage, and finding new health coverage with a pre-existing diagnosis can be difficult and expensive.

Document all contact with the human resources department and insurance company, and get everything in writing, such as permission to go out-of-network or referrals to specialists. Include date, time, name of the person with whom you spoke, issues discussed, and resolution or plan. Keep all of this information organized in a filing system, and always keep copies of any materials you send to the insurance company. If the patient needs to dispute coverage decisions, all of this tedious documentation will be invaluable, as it will save time and energy in the long run.

82. What if insurance denies a claim?

If you think that the insurance company has denied a claim that should have been covered or is discontinuing coverage, first contact the patient's insurance company and/or human resources department if health insurance is provided via her workplace. Sometimes simple changes need to be made to fix the problem. For example, claims can be rejected for reasons such as having your incorrect birth date or social security number (SSN) in the computer system or on a form.

If an initial telephone inquiry does not work, write a letter to the insurance carrier, clearly stating the claim number, the date of service, the correct personal information of the patient (policy and group numbers, SSN, birth date, name, and address), and the reason you believe the claim should have been approved. Be direct but pleasant in your tone, and keep a copy of the letter. The carrier may request additional medical information before covering certain tests or treatments, and sometimes sending additional documentation or having the doctor contact the carrier can resolve these issues. If you have exhausted all other options, you can contact your state's insurance commissioner or hire a lawyer who specializes in insurance disputes.

Recent legislation at the state and national level exists to protect patients, in some limited ways, from insurance coverage lapses due to medical diagnosis and unfair claim rejections. Private insurance companies and **health maintenance organizations** (HMOs) are

Health Maintenance Organization (HMO)

an organization providing health care to enrolled members through a network of member doctors and other healthcare providers.

most likely regulated by your State Department of Insurance or State Department of Health. See the Appendix for specific references to learn more about these laws and how to seek assistance, including the National Coalition for Cancer Survivorship's publication entitled, *What Cancer Survivors Need to Know About Health Insurance.*

PART EIGHT

Work Concerns

What is the difference between Social Security Disability (SSD), Supplemental Security Income (SSI), Social Security (SS), and public assistance (welfare)? How can a patient apply?

How should patients negotiate for sick leave or disability leave from work? Also, how do I negotiate for time off from work to be with my family member for medical appointments and to help her at home?

Will my partner be able to continue working during radiation therapy and chemotherapy?

More ...

83. What is the difference between Social Security Disability (SSD), Supplemental Security Income (SSI), Social Security (SS), and public assistance (welfare)? How can a patient apply?

There are many government programs, particularly at the state and federal level, which can assist with health care coverage and financial assistance for eligible recipients. There are also types of private insurance policies, such as long-term care insurance or private disability insurance, and many other government programs not discussed here. However, some of the most common programs, along with brief descriptions of each program, are provided below. For more comprehensive information on **public assistance**, or for information on programs not mentioned here, refer to the resources provided in this section and at the end of this book.

- *Social Security Disability* (SSD; U.S. Social Security Administration; *www.ssa.gov*): Provides monthly income to disabled workers and their families based on prior payroll contribution and disabled status.
- If person becomes disabled before the age he or she is eligible for full Social Security benefits, he or she can receive SSD payments after 6 months if he or she has:
  1. enough Social Security credits, and
  2. a physical or mental impairment that is expected to prevent the person from doing substantial work for 1 year or more, or a condition that is expected to result in death.
- *Social Security* (SS; U.S. Social Security Administration; *www.ssa.gov*): Social Security provides monthly payments to persons age 65 and over and

---

Public assistance

federally run program to provide cash benefits (food stamps, Welfare) for persons with a low-income to purchase food and clothing and to pay for housing.

surviving family members (after the recipient's death, including dependents). Eligibility entails contributing to Social Security during a person's previous work history, and the amount of payment is based on a formula that considers the amount contributed during that history.

- *Veterans Benefits*: If a person is a U.S. veteran, contact the Department of Veterans Affairs to investigate **veterans' benefits** for which he or she is eligible (including possible financial assistance and/or medical care). Qualified veterans can also receive discounts on prescription drugs.

- *Supplemental Security Income* (SSI; U.S. Social Security Administration, *www.ssa.gov*): Provides monthly income to eligible people over the age of 65, or to blind or disabled people, with low income, few assets, and/or limited formal work history. SSI may also provide benefits for people waiting for SSD payments to begin. U.S. citizenship is required, with few exceptions. If you are eligible for SSI, you may also be eligible for Medicaid, food stamps (see below) and other assistance.

- *Public Assistance* (welfare/food stamps; individual states' Department of Social Services): Provides cash benefits to low-income persons for food, clothing, and shelter. Benefits vary depending on assets, income, rent/mortgage, living arrangements, work expenses, and other special needs. Some states require recipients to work, and if they are unable to work due to illness, the agencies may require a physician's examination as confirmation. Food stamps provide a monthly allotment of coupons for low-income households to purchase food at grocery stores and meals in some restaurants.

Work Concerns

Veterans' benefits
financial and/or medical care and discounted prescription drugs that may be available for U.S. veterans.

84. Whom should I tell at work that my family member has cancer?

Telling people at work may have benefits, but disclosure can also have some potential drawbacks. Many people have close friends at work, and talking to these colleagues may provide them emotional support and opportunity to talk about their experiences. You may find that people you know have gone through similar experiences and can provide some good advice. However, many family members have told us that sometimes "advice" can be unsolicited, unhelpful, and sometimes overwhelming. Family members may tell a lot of people in the beginning of the diagnosis, and then later regret the widespread disclosure because it seems like the "whole world" knows their personal business. It can then be hard to simply escape thinking about and discussing the cancer, and to focus on work.

If you do want to disclose, you may want to consider telling only the people who need to know. For example, it may (or may not) be necessary to tell your supervisor or human resources staff in order to receive time off to attend medical appointments or care for the patient. Telling one or two trusted friends, specifying that you want to keep the diagnosis confidential, may be a way to obtain needed support and attempt to maintain control over what people know about the cancer diagnosis. You can also be selective in what you disclose. For example, you may say that your family member has cancer, but you do not have to talk about the specifics, such as stage of the disease, treatments, or the details about how the patient is doing. Furthermore, sometimes people at work will know the patient, or in smaller communities where "everyone knows everyone," it is important to consider your loved one's feelings about disclosure as well. Together, with the patient and other family and friends, talk about who is to be told, and what they will be told.

85. How should patients negotiate for sick leave or disability leave from work? Also, how do I negotiate for time off from work to be with my family member for medical appointments and to help her at home?

If your loved one is currently working or plans to resume work and she believes the treatment schedule will interfere with working, she can ask her employer about flexibility in hours to accommodate treatment and appointments. Additionally, she should inquire about temporary disability insurance, continued health care coverage, and medical or family leave. Employees who have accrued enough sick time may not have to dip into these benefits. We have also seen patients bring work with them to the hospital and, when possible, continue a productive work schedule.

As a primary caregiver for an ill person, you may also be entitled to time off from your workplace in order to provide care to the patient. First, you may want to speak with your supervisor to discuss the possibility of a flexible work schedule to accommodate medical appointments, and so forth. For example, instead of working nine to five, maybe medical appointments can be scheduled in the mornings, and you can arrive to work late and work late. This way, you may be able to maintain your full work schedule, keeping your full income and benefits.

However, often people cannot alter their work schedule this way. You should assess your employer's policy on taking personal days, vacation days, and possibly sick leave to care for an ill family member. Some companies have a pool of employee-donated sick hours for those who need them. Family medical leave for more extended periods also may be possible. According to the Family Medical Leave Act, eligible employees are able to take unpaid leave from work for up to 12 weeks and be guaranteed the same or similar position and pay when they return. Before quoting this law to your employers, however, investigate how it applies to your circumstance. Search the ACS Web site (*www.cancer.org*) for specific topics or consult the U.S. Department of Labor for details (see the Appendix).

Make sure that you are able to continue health care insurance coverage.

If you take family leave, be aware that your employer is not required to hold your same job, only a comparable one, and that you may not have the same benefits, such as medical coverage, during your leave. These issues are important to consider, especially if the patient is receiving health insurance benefits from your workplace benefits. Therefore, make sure that you are able to continue health care insurance coverage. This will entail either you or your employer paying the premium. You may also spread out the days away from the job; for example, you may want to take off two days a week, instead of taking leave all at once. Investigate your employer's policies by speaking with your human resources department and/or your supervisor.

86. I have to go to work for financial reasons, but I feel so bad about leaving my husband to go to medical appointments without me. How can I do my job and not feel so guilty?

Mark's comment:

Your commitments to your day-to-day life can't end because someone you love is sick. If you stopped working to take care of him or her all the time, you'd both starve, which isn't an improvement on the current situation! Sometimes practical matters just have to come first, and to heck with feeling guilty about it—it's the way it has to be, and that's the end of it.

Family and friends are often torn between providing support and care for the patient and their other life duties, such as work. This is particularly true if there are financial concerns, since this adds to the pressure and sense of conflict between providing financial support and providing care. First of all, talk to your husband about how you feel, and ask him if he wants or needs someone with him at every appointment. Sometimes caregivers feel an overwhelming sense of responsibility to be with patients at every minute, and, ironically, patients sometimes want a bit of time to themselves but they don't say anything for fear of hurting family members' feelings.

Most importantly, you need to acknowledge that you cannot physically and emotionally "do everything." If the patient does want companionship or assistance during an inpatient hospitalization, for example, you may ask other family or friends to take "shifts" being with your loved one during your work day. You can then schedule your shift for evenings and weekends. For outpatient appointments, ask these people to assist with driving your husband to and from appointments (if he is unable to drive) or visit him during longer chemotherapy treatments. This plan also provides opportunities for other friends and family members to spend quality time with your husband, and fosters feelings that they are contributing to his care. If you do not have others who can assist, and you can afford it, consider hiring a private aide or nurse to supplement your care (at home or in the hospital).

On an emotional level, guilt is a feeling that arises when someone believes he or she is doing something to harm someone, or believes he or she is not doing enough to prevent harm. Loved ones have told us that they feel pressure to do everything for the patient because they fear that if they do not do everything, the cancer will come back, or worse, their loved one will die. As long as your husband is not in danger, you need to establish realistic limits and understand that you are neither responsible for your husband's cancer, nor are you going to make the cancer worse by setting realistic limits and doing necessary life tasks, such as going to work. In fact, sometimes family members do too much for patients, increasing dependence and reducing helpful physical activity. If your husband is physically capable, it may be good to support his independence and his sense of control by encouraging him to continue to do household chores and/or other activities by himself.

87. Will my partner be able to continue working during radiation therapy and chemotherapy?

The choice to continue working during treatments is a personal one. Radiation therapy sometimes requires being at the hospital or clinic an hour a day, and chemotherapy can also require regular visits to the hospital, posing a time constraint. Ideal times for treatment cannot always be coordinated with a person's work schedule. In addition, although the treatments themselves are usually painless, patients may experience various side effects because of the toxic nature of the treatments. In other words, sometimes the substances or treatments that are given with the intent to kill the cancer can make a person feel sick as well.

For example, some patients experience diarrhea and fatigue as treatment side effects. Although these symptoms can be minor, they can sometimes become more bothersome, particularly when radiation therapy and chemotherapy are combined. Your partner's choice of how much work she plans to accomplish should be based on the type of work, the convenience of the hospital relative to her daily activities, your loved one's ability to tolerate treatments, and other issues, such as financial considerations and her employer's flexibility.

The truth is that no one knows how your partner will react to treatments until after starting them. If possible, she may want to begin with a more limited work schedule (meaning less than what she thinks she can handle) and then add hours onto her schedule, depending on how she feels and how high her energy level is. Not only will committing to fewer hours prevent her from falling short of expectations at work, but it will also be good psychologically. It always feels good to do more than expected (when possible) rather then less than expected. With an altered work schedule, many patients are able to continue working during treatment. If your partner decides that she cannot work or chooses not to work for other reasons during her treatments (such as to spend more time with family and friends), she may be eligible for short-term disability through her workplace and/or Social Security Disability (see Question 83).

88. Is my family member protected from workplace discrimination?

Legislation, such as the Americans with Disabilities Act (ADA), protects disabled people from certain types of workplace discrimination. A person with cancer or a history of cancer may be protected under the ADA. However, the ADA is complex, applies only to companies that meet specific criteria, and has other limitations. Other federal laws (such as the Federal Rehabilitation Act, the Family and Medical Leave Act, and the Employee Retirement and Income Security Act) and state laws also exist to protect employees with health issues. Aspects of these laws likewise pertain to health insurance coverage, particularly the Comprehensive Omnibus Budget Reconciliation Act (COBRA), which makes group insurance policies provided by certain employers available to employees, even those who have quit, been terminated, or work fewer hours. To learn more about work concerns and legislation, consult a social worker or purchase the National Coalition for Cancer Survivorship's publication, *Working It Out: Your Employment Rights As a Cancer Survivor* (see the Appendix for contact information).

PART NINE

Emotional Reactions & Practical Concerns About Death and Dying

Is thinking about death bad luck?

The doctors say that there is nothing more they can do to treat my wife's cancer. What do I do now? Just give up?

Is making "quality of life" the goal going to shorten my husband's life?

More . . .

89. Is thinking about death bad luck? Although he doesn't talk much about it, I know my husband has been thinking about death and dying since the doctors first suspected he might have cancer. How much is normal?

Mark's comment:

People who think of death as a bad thing don't understand that it can be a release sometimes—if your loved one's body is so severely damaged by disease, the spirit is relieved of that hurt when it's set free by death. But thinking about death is not the same thing as obsessing about death. If death becomes an obsession, if you think about it and worry about it all the time, then you may need to get counseling.

When someone is faced with the news that he or she has cancer, frequent thoughts of death are common. Death is something that, at least in the United States and many Western cultures, people often try to forget about; they simply deny that it exists. A cancer diagnosis cuts right through this denial, and fears of mortality flood through. Some people are more prepared for this realization; others are not. For those who are less prepared, this may be the first time in their lives that they have truly realized they are mortal. Thoughts of death may include the following:

1. Thinking about one's own impending death and what it will be like

2. Remembering past experiences with death and losses

3. Paying more attention to death in the news or books

4. Talking more about it to family, friends, or religious advisors

5. Worrying about pain and other medical aspects about the dying process

Ironically, understanding one's own beliefs about death can be helpful to coping. In order to understand himself better, your husband should pay attention to when he thinks about death, what he thinks about, and how he feels about these thoughts. Let him know that if he wants to discuss these issues, he should find someone with whom he can talk openly about death and dying. You may not be that someone, at least right now, for various reasons. He simply may not be ready to talk with you about it, or you may not be ready to hear it. Don't take it personally if he chooses not to discuss these thoughts with you now. It may take time and practice before he is able to discuss these things with someone very close. Also, people close to patients sometimes misinterpret discussions of death as "giving up" or find it too much to handle, in which case someone more objective to speak to, such as a religious advisor, a doctor or nurse, or a counselor, may make it less stressful for both of you.

Thinking about death neither makes it come faster nor is it bad luck. However, if your husband finds himself thinking about death and dying for long periods of time (for most of the day, many days in a row), or if he is thinking about taking steps to end his life, contact his doctor or a mental health professional immediately. Call 911 if he has plans to hurt himself or others. Depression and other psychological issues can make thoughts of death overwhelming.

Thinking about death neither makes it come faster nor is it bad luck.

Additionally, people who are experiencing various physical symptoms or side effects may misinterpret these experiences, believing that they are actually dying when, in fact, they are not. Pain and other factors altering quality of life are common and may precede thoughts of wanting to die. However, when these medical problems are solved, thoughts of death or wishes to die usually subside as well. Therefore, if your husband is comfortable, encourage him to *talk* about his thoughts and feelings about dying with his family and/or with the medical team so that he understands these thoughts are normal. Sharing feelings can be helpful to him and may also help you, the rest of the family, and the medical team better understand what your husband is experiencing. When all of you understand him better, you can help him more effectively in his time of distress.

90. The doctors say that there is nothing more they can do to treat my wife's cancer. What do I do now? Just give up?

This time period is often filled with important decisions. Make sure that you fully understand what the doctor is telling you. He or she may not be able to give you a specific prognosis, but make sure that you are clear about what the doctor is saying about your wife's condition. Why, exactly, is there nothing left to do? If your wife is interested in getting more treatment, be sure to ask about any other possible treatments available, including experimental treatments. Remember that you always have the option of seeking a medical opinion from another physician.

After investigating the options, your wife may decide to discontinue treatment, which is sometimes the hardest decision for patients, and physicians, to make. Physicians use different words ("palliation," "**support-**

ive care," and "**comfort care**") to represent a shift from focusing on curing the cancer to treating the symptoms of cancer during the later stages of the disease process. Active palliative care sometimes involves chemotherapy, radiation therapy, or even surgery to help alleviate such symptoms. Supportive care and comfort care also refer to symptom management, often with the use of medications, and may include hospice care (see Question 92).

Ending treatment that has not cured the cancer is often a shock for patients and family members. For example, you may feel hopeless, overwhelmed, and/or angry, and these feelings may be directed at the doctor for not being able to cure your loved one, or at the patient—or yourself—for not "fighting hard enough." These are all normal reactions. Emotions such as sadness, loss, and despair sometimes follow. Other people may have prepared themselves for when this time was coming and may be more accepting of the impending death (particularly if they discussed these issues beforehand with their support system members).

During this time, people in the later stages of the illness often focus on making their last days as positive as possible. If you and your loved one are in this situation, there are some questions to ask her, the answers to which may help both of you better understand how each of you feels and what her wishes are at this time. Ask your wife, "Do you want to be in the hospital during your last days? At home? At a hospice facility? Do you want to be pain free? Whom do you want to be with you? What do you want to do before you die? Express your feelings for your loved ones? Make amends with someone? Pray and focus on your spiritu-

Supportive care
focused on treating the symptoms of disease in the later stages of the terminal disease process.

Comfort care
focused on treating the symptoms of disease in the later stages of the disease process.

Emotional Reactions & Practical Concerns

ality? Do you have any specific religious tasks you want to complete? Do you believe in an afterlife? If so, what do you imagine? Is it fearful or comforting to you?"

Answering these questions is difficult. Discussing them with others may be more so. This is a time when many people look back on their lives, focusing on their relationships, the meaning of life and death, and possibly their relationship with God. Your loved one may struggle psychologically with understanding and coping with her death. She may also struggle to help your family cope with death. You, on the other hand, may or may not understand all her decisions. Your loved one may have philosophical questions that cannot be answered, or she may feel anxious about leaving loved ones. All of these issues and more may arise. Often, meeting with a chaplain or spiritual advisor, social worker, or the doctor can help patients and family find answers to questions and reduce distress about common concerns that arise during the later stages of life.

91. Even though my husband is still alive, I find myself thinking about my life after he dies. Somehow, this doesn't seem right—is it wrong to have these kinds of thoughts?

Some people, when faced with the impending loss of a loved one, prepare themselves by imagining what life will be like after the loss and how they will react. They can even experience emotions similar to those they would feel if their loved one had already passed away. This preparation, referred to as **anticipatory grief** by

Anticipatory grief

beginning to experience the loss of someone before the person actually dies.

some, may serve to lessen the distress of bereavement later on and to facilitate the adjustment process.

You should not judge yourself for having these kinds of thoughts and feelings. But be aware if they are affecting the way you think of your husband in the present here and now and how you act toward him. There is the possibility of separating yourself too early from your loved one through anticipatory grief. Your husband still needs you, and there are still meaningful opportunities to experience and celebrate the value of your life together and your relationship with one another. Preparing yourself should not leave you emotionally distant from him.

92. What is hospice?

When discussing end-of-life decisions, medical professionals may use the word "hospice" and sometimes assume that you know what this means. Hospice is a type of care focusing on improving or maintaining quality of life, as opposed to extending life, when a person is no longer seeking treatment to cure his or her cancer. Hospice can be provided either at home or at an inpatient facility. Hospice focuses on symptom management, and this means alleviating the pain, nausea, and general distress that is common for people during the dying process. Hospices are often staffed by nurses, doctors (who can adjust pain medication), social workers, psychiatrists, chaplains, and other support staff. You may read more about hospice from the resource list in the back of this book. The American Cancer Society has very helpful information its Web site, as does the National Hospice and Palliative Care Organization (NHPCO). If you believe the time is right, you may ask your doctor about hospice care if he or she does not initiate this discussion with you.

If hospice care is appropriate, and you and your loved one choose this type of care, hospice services will provide support to both patient and caregivers. We have had a few patients or caregivers state they were afraid of hospice care, thinking that it meant that they had given up all hope. Do not think of hospice in this way. Accepting hospice care will not hasten your loved one's death. His or her symptoms will be better managed, so that you can spend more quality time with him or her and enjoy the time you do have left as much as possible. We have seen many patients choose hospice care, which relieved their symptoms so well that they were able to continue with daily activities, such as going out and socializing, which they otherwise probably would not have been able to do. Also, a person does not have to be in the final stages of dying in order to be eligible for hospice, particularly home hospice. In fact, the earlier a patient receives these services, the more likely the patient and the family will benefit. Furthermore, the patient may be able to receive palliative treatments (such as chemotherapy or radiation therapy) and still be eligible for hospice. Ask your social worker or doctor to investigate this option.

93. By making "quality of life" the goal, is this going to shorten my husband's life?

"Quality of life" can mean different things to different people. For some, simply being alive is worthwhile. For others, they expect a certain level of ability to function, both physically and mentally, in order to retain their sense of dignity. When the medical team shifts its focus to comfort care, saying that there is little prospect for curing the cancer, there may still be other treatments they can employ to both fight back the cancer, at least temporarily, and/or relieve the symptoms of the disease. In some cases, managing a person's painful or uncomfortable symptoms, in fact, results in *living longer* than if these treatments were not provided. Therefore, focusing on enhancing quality of life will not shorten a person's life.

The decision of whether to pursue such treatments, however, becomes more complicated when the treatments carry with them the risk or likelihood of adverse side effects. What if this chemotherapy makes the patient feel sicker even though the growth of the tumor is slowed? What if whole brain radiation therapy results in memory loss and confusion even though it relieves the patient's headaches? In these cases, electing not to have the treatments can result in a shorter time left to live. However, if there is a trade-off between quality of life versus possibly extending life, one can only decide for oneself where the tipping point lies and when to forego further treatment. People with cancer individually choose their own paths to follow. Helping them to define what quality of life means to them, to articulate their hopes and fears about the final stage of their life, and to make sure they are getting enough accurate information about their options to make an informed decision provides important support.

94. What is a health care proxy and living will?

The death process in the United States has been dramatically altered in the face of new medical technology that saves and sustains life. With these advancements come difficult decisions about when to use, and withdraw, such treatments. Even with the best care available today, there may come a time when your loved one's cancer has progressed beyond conventional treatments. During this time, because of cancer spread to the liver, lungs, or brain, he may not be mentally able to make decisions regarding his own care. Family members (or another person previously designated) will then be asked to make medical decisions on the patient's behalf.

In order to facilitate the decision-making process and address the communication, emotional, and sometimes ethical issues that can arise, a legal system was established, which varies from state to state. The general term for the documents is an **advance directive**, placed in the patient's medical record, which describes his wishes regarding various life-sustaining medical interventions in the event that the patient cannot communicate his wishes directly. This allows a person to take control of his care and preserve his dignity in the event of complicated situations.

Patients can assign a health care proxy to help make medical decisions if they are too debilitated to do so themselves. A **health care proxy** (sometimes called a medical durable power of attorney or a health care agent) is an officially designated medical decision-maker (identified by a document or verbal identification) who acts on the patient's behalf if he becomes unable to make medical decisions (due either to temporary situations or to enduring ones, such as being permanently comatose).

Many states have family consent laws, establishing a clear succession of family members to be identified as

Advance directive

a document in the patient's record describing his or her wishes regarding various life-sustaining interventions in the event the patient cannot communicate directly.

Health care proxy

a legal document (also called medical durable power of attorney or health care agent) designating a family member, guardian, or friend as the decision-maker about medical treatment for a patient.

surrogate medical decision makers, if a patient has not otherwise named and documented a proxy. If you live in such a state, it is particularly important that the patient legally identify a health care proxy if he does not want the state-designated family member to be his surrogate decision maker. For example, the laws usually do not recognize non-married partners (even for couples who have been together for a long time) as part of the succession. Instead, a parent or adult child, or a more distant relative could be designated as the surrogate and make crucial decisions about a person's medical care.

For this reason, it is often best if the proxy is someone with whom the patient has a close relationship and who is aware of his feelings about extreme life support measures in the setting of a terminal disease. In states that do not have family consent laws, such as New York, it is particularly important that patients have identified a health care proxy and discussed their wishes with that person, since a family member may not have the legal right to make decisions on their behalf without having been formally identified as the health care proxy.

Patients can develop a **living will** describing their wishes regarding specific medical interventions toward the end of life and can be very specific regarding individual therapies that the person either desires or does not desire to have. The use of prolonged ventilation with a respirator, the placement of tubes for artificial feeding, and the choice for cardiopulmonary resuscitation (CPR) are common topics for clarification in a living will. The information is documented in the patient's medical record and informs the decisions to

Living will

legal document that specifies a patient's wishes in the event he or she becomes mentally incapacitated.

manage his care should the need arise. However, it is still important for a patient to identify a surrogate decision-maker/health care proxy and discuss his or her values and wishes with the surrogate and physician. Living wills can help guide doctor and family decisions, but rarely are they specific enough to apply to all possible medical circumstances that may arise.

95. What is a DNR order?

Do not resuscitate order (DNR)

can be a component of advance directive and a living will; specifies the medical steps to be taken in the event the patient is found to be minimally responsive with minimal life signs.

DNR stands for "**do not resuscitate**" and is a common component of advance directives, including a living will. A DNR order dictates the steps to be taken if a patient is found to be minimally responsive with minimal life signs. It mandates whether medical steps, such as intubation or cardiopulmonary resuscitation (CPR), should be administered if a patient goes into cardiac arrest. The Patient Self-Determination Act enacted in 1991 gives all patients the right to accept or refuse resuscitative efforts in accordance with state laws or statutes.

The DNR order is a difficult issue for patients, families, and healthcare providers. It is a potentially emotional topic and decision, and may generate conflicts between/among the people involved if there is disagreement about the right course of action. For example, some patients and family members may believe that, under all circumstances, all efforts should be made to prolong life and would therefore refuse a DNR order. Other people may believe that death should occur more naturally, without life support and other medical interventions, and agree to a DNR order. Caregivers and family members may certainly express their beliefs; however, individual feelings and conflict should be tempered by an understanding of the patient's true wishes.

To protect themselves with advance directives, patients should be encouraged to initiate a discussion of their wishes with their healthcare team and their family, and particularly with their physician(s) and their healthcare proxy—not only so that their wishes are upheld, but also so that the doctor and the proxy understand their wishes. Having these difficult, but meaningful conversations in advance removes a lot of the burden of making these decisions from the family and friends. They will not have to guess or speculate about the patient's wishes.

Additionally, it is important to understand that *a DNR order does not mean the withdrawal of care*. Patients will not be segregated into a separate section of the hospital and neglected while "waiting to die." Their medical needs such as pain control or other supportive medical care will be provided. The DNR order comes into play only if a patient requires resuscitation.

Nancy's comment:

A DNR order assumes that the patient will die in the hospital. In fact, dying at home is the desire of most terminally ill people. For this reason, a copy of the DNR, health care proxy and/or living will statements should be kept in a visible and accessible place in the patient's home. Should the caregiver or someone else find the patient dying or dead in the house, you should know that a 911 call will bring EMT personnel whose task is to revive the patient and provide life support while transporting him or her to the emergency room—exactly the opposite of what the DNR and most living wills are intended to convey. Even if the patient is taken to a hospital that has treated him or her before—which isn't guaranteed in an emergency—ER personnel don't necessarily have access to patient's chart in the doctor's office or hospital records and probably will not check for a DNR order. If the caregiver doesn't have a health care proxy document in hand and can't immediately produce the living will or DNR documents, he or she will be unable to insist that the hospital personnel do not attempt resuscitation. So it's very important to make sure that these records are kept in a prominent place if the patient doesn't want resuscitation or heroic measures.

96. Even though we talked about it, I don't know if I can make a "life or death decision" for my husband. Would it be so terrible just to let nature take its course?

Surrogate decision makers who agree to a DNR order and/or to stop life-sustaining medical intervention may feel guilt or that they are "giving up," even though they are acting according to the patient's previously stated wishes and/or in the best interests of the patient. Other difficult decisions for surrogates including asking for more pain medication for dying patients with extremely advanced disease, since the amount of medication required to alleviate their symptoms can make them less alert and, in rare circumstances, hasten a person's death by a short amount of time. This can be extremely distressing to the people making medical decisions for their loved ones.

People who do not react well to a crisis may respond in two basic ways. One is to make rash decisions based on blind emotion rather that reasoned thought. The other is to wait and do nothing, which is often the result of "paralysis by analysis." The latter choice is more common and may seem reasonable given what we have previously said about collecting as much information as possible in order to make an informed decision. However, by waiting, you may be prolonging the patient's status in a state of indignity. Furthermore, prolonging treatment for a patient who previously stated that she did not want to be treated or be on life-support in this condition is not ethical. If you come to an impasse, try to limit yourself time-wise: Ask the doctors how long you have to make the decision, and if it seems reasonable, try to stick to it. Talk to involved family members and others whom you think can help you make the best decision.

For some people, the underlying issues are that they just do not want the responsibility and/or they simply cannot bear to let go of their loved one emotionally. Remember that your decision as a proxy needs to be based on the patient's preferences as you best understand them. If these preferences are not clear in your mind, then speak with other people who might have insight into them: friends, family, and the doctors. Patients will often have a discussion of this sort with the medical team when family isn't present precisely because they don't wish to upset them. Both of us have had in-depth conversations with patients about their wishes regarding life-sustaining treatment and have helped patients relate these wishes to their surrogate. If you do agree to a DNR order or an increase in a medication dosage, you probably won't be asked to sign anything. This is because these orders come from the physician, not from you. It is they who are directing the course of care, and thus sharing the responsibility for any decision with you. If you have concerns or

Emotional Reactions & Practical Concerns

Prolonging treatment for a patient who previously stated that she did not want to be treated or be on life-support in this condition is not ethical.

questions about end-of-life care issues, speak with the physician. Furthermore, ethics consultants, patient advocates, or social workers are available for extra guidance. If the situation reaches an impasse, all hospitals are required to have an ethics committee where you, the doctors, and other involved people can meet to discuss solutions.

Remember, by stopping life-sustaining treatment, you are not killing the patient. The cancer and/or underlying medical condition is what causes the person's death.

97. What do I do now that my loved one is dying?

Nancy's comment:

As family members gather to say goodbye and sit by the patient, a living eulogy can allow the patient to feel that he or she has lived a valued and important life. Remembering and sharing memories about the good times accomplishes this task, and sharing even the tough times helps the dying with the difficulty of saying goodbye. Even when lives are fraught with misadventure, everyone has some good that can be encouraged, discussed, and honored.

You may now have reached the point where your loved one is "actively dying," a process which, without heroic medical intervention, will result in the body ceasing to function. If you haven't already done so, ask the doctors what you can expect to happen physically. As difficult as it is, information on the dying process will help you to prepare for the final stage of your loved one's life. Knowing in advance what symptoms can occur, such as pain, shortness of breath, or breath sounds, gives you the opportunity to discuss with the medical team the treatments to make your loved one most comfortable. Being informed also helps ensure that these treatments are provided in a timely manner later, particularly during times of crisis.

Managing the practical aspects of care for a dying person, whether in the hospital with the medical team or at home through a hospice program, can be looked at partly as another test of your problem-solving skills. But the greater part is the emotional challenge of managing your fear and grief in the face of imminent loss. On the one hand, you are trying to provide your loved one a safe passage. You are looking after this person's physical comfort, reassuring your loved one that he or she is not alone, maintaining his or her sense of dignity, assisting him or her in defining and expressing whatever thoughts that he or she might have—and want to share—about the meaning and value of life in his or her final days. On the other hand, you are saying goodbye to each other, beginning that process that allows both of you to let go of one another.

The hard part is staying close to the dying person—that is, remaining practically and emotionally involved—but knowing when to give him or her permission to go, so that he or she does not feel either guilty about dying or abandoned by you. The actual goodbye can be phrased in different ways, but as Ira Byock, a well-known expert on dying suggests, there are five things that people may want to say in one way or another: "Forgive me;" "I forgive you;" "Thank you;" "I love you;" and finally, "Good-bye."

98. What do I do, now that my loved one has died?

What you have to do afterward depends on whether the death occurs in the hospital or at home. In the hospital, the body will be moved to the morgue and kept there until you have made arrangements for its disposition. This doesn't have to be decided immediately. Although there are public health laws that limit the number of days the body can remain there, most hospitals give families 3 days to a week to get in touch with a funeral home or some other service. Funeral homes will then contact the hospital and make all the arrangements for transporting the body. If the death occurs at home, you do not have to call the police, but you should call the hospice program or the primary physician. You can then contact the funeral home or crematorium, which will then arrange to have the body transported to their facility.

After you've informed family members and friends of what's happened, you will also need to contact the attorney, financial planner, and/or accountant to begin settling your loved one's estate. Other business matters that will need attending to include contacting the bank to close accounts and notifying the Social Security Administration, Department of Veterans Affairs, insurance companies, and former employers and/or unions, in order to apply for any benefits that you or other family members might be entitled to. These agencies will ask you for copies of the death certificate for verification, so be sure to obtain several duplicates, either through the funeral director or the health department.

99. What are the tasks of grieving, and what does it feel like?

According to J. William Worden, who has written extensively about grief, there are four principal tasks that are essential to the mourning process: 1) accepting the reality of the loss; 2) working through the pain of grief; 3) adjusting to life without the deceased; and 4) "emotionally relocating the deceased and moving on, " which does not mean forgetting the deceased, but rather finding "an appropriate place" for them "in their emotional lives—a place that will enable [those left behind] to go on living effectively in the world."

Grieving is painful. People in grief can experience feelings of sadness, anger, guilt, and/or anxiety, as well as physical sensations, such as hollowness in the stomach or tightness in the chest and tearfulness, among others. There can be a variety of changes in the way they think and act: confusion, preoccupation, longing for the deceased, searching and calling out, sleep and appetite disturbances, social withdrawal, and sometimes restless hyperactivity. These reactions will normally diminish and pass with time. Talking with your family and friends, a member of the clergy, or a grief counselor can help you manage your grief.

In Worden's view, mourning the loss of a close relationship requires at least a year, possibly two, though this varies greatly depending on the individual and cultural background. Mourning is completed when the

[1]Worden JW. *Grief Counseling and Grief Therapy: A Handbook for the Mental Health Practitioner,* 3rd Edition. Springer Publishing Co., 2001.

Emotional Reactions & Practical Concerns

bereaved person can think of the deceased without pain and can "reinvest his or her emotions back into life and in the living." If you experience grief that is so intense that it leaves you feeling overwhelmed or unable to cope, or lasts for an overly long period of time, your grieving process may require the intervention of a grief specialist, to help you work toward completion of the tasks of mourning. Long periods of grief can lead to clinical depression, so talk with a professional if you are concerned about the depth or breadth of your grief process.

As a caregiver, you may feel relief now that your caregiving responsibilities have come to an end upon the death of your loved one. For some, these feelings can lead to further feelings of guilt beyond those normally experienced by survivors. Others become anxious, because in addition to the loss of their loved one, they are losing their roles as family member and caregiver that had deeply defined them—and their lives—for a long period of time. You are now embarking on your own journey of healing. Be kind to yourself, use the techniques and strategies we've provided in this book to help you cope, and don't forget to reach out to others to help you find your place in the world again.

100. Where can I find more information?

The Appendix that follows contains resources that will be helpful to both patients and caregivers. Although not all publications or organizations are represented here, the resources in this list are excellent starting points.

General Resources

American Cancer Society (ACS)
American Cancer Society National Home Office
1599 Clifton Road
Atlanta, GA 30329
(800) ACS-2345
www.cancer.org
ACS is an excellent resource for a wide-range of issues, including information
on the medical aspects of cancer, coping and family issues, making medical
decisions and much more. In addition to their superb Web site, they also publish a variety books and pamphlets (see a sampling of titles below), facilitate
support groups and lectures run by local ACS offices (you can search the Web
site or call for program details), and are involved in advocacy and government
policies issues. In some locations, they can provide limited financial assistance
to people in financial need undergoing treatment for cancer. Some information is available in Spanish. Publications include the following:
Caring for the Patient with Cancer at Home: A Guide for Patients and Families
Our Mom Has Cancer
American Cancer Society's Health Eating Cookbook, 2nd edition
Caregiving
Cancer in the Family
Couples Confronting Cancer
Because . . . Someone I Love Has Cancer

American Society of Clinical Oncology
1900 Duke Street, Suite 200
Alexandria, VA 22314
(703) 299-0150
www.asco.org
www.peoplelivingwithcancer.org
"The American Society of Clinical Oncology is a 501(c)(3) nonprofit organization that represents more than 19,000 cancer professionals worldwide. ASCO

offers scientific and educational programs as well as a wide range of other initiatives intended to foster the exchange of information about cancer." (Web site) A section of the Web site is dedicated to "People Living with Cancer" (*www.people livingwithcancer.org*) and provides information on cancer prevention and treatment, as well as other useful resources, such as online discussion groups, and specific information on types of oncologists plus tips on how to select the best oncologist for you. Also provides information about specific drugs, a medical dictionary, and issues related to coping. Online "live" chats with medical providers, as well as information on genetic testing and clinical trials, are featured.

Association of Oncology Social Workers (AOSW)
1211 Locust Street
Philadelphia, PA 19107
(215) 599-6093
(215) 545-8107 (fax)
info@aosw.org
www.aosw.org
"The Association of Oncology Social Work (AOSW) is a nonprofit, international organization dedicated to the enhancement of psychosocial services to people with cancer and their families" (Web site). The organization is primarily a professional organization for oncology social workers; the Web site does provide information and links to resources which may be helpful to patients and their families.

Association of Cancer Online Resources, Inc. (ACOR)
173 Duane Street
Suite 3A
New York NY 10013-3334
(212) 226-5525
www.acor.org
ACOR provides information and links to other online resources via its Web site as well as Internet mailing lists. One useful feature of the Web site is found under the "Publications" link, where you can search for books on specific cancer-related topics (click on "Cancer Bibliography") and other features, such as Medline updates on the latest scientific abstracts about specific cancer types (click on "The Latest Scientific Abstracts" and then choose your topic).

Cancer Care, Inc.

275 7th Avenue

New York, NY 10001

(212) 712-8400 (administration)

(212) 712-8080 (services)

www.cancercare.org

"Cancer Care is a national non-profit organization whose mission is to provide free professional help to people with all cancers through counseling, education, information and referral and direct financial assistance" (Web site). You may find the reliable online information very helpful and may choose to investigate the online and telephone support groups and lectures in addition to the many other resources and services this organization provides. Much information is provided in Spanish as well as English, and counseling locations are currently available throughout the NY/NJ/CT tri-state area.

CancerLinks

www.cancerlinks.org (online only)

This site is simply a list of links specific to various types of cancer. The site is constantly updated providing the latest list of links available. This is a great starting place to begin an online search about cancer.

Cancer Research Institute

681 Fifth Avenue

New York, NY 10022

(800) 99-CANCER (800-992-2623)

www.cancerresearch.org

This site focuses on scientific research and funding; however, the link, *www.cancerresearch.org/hbintro.html,* does provide a simple list of common questions and answers regarding concerns about cancer and a resource directory, which includes financial support and home care referral sources.

Cancer Research Foundation of America

1600 Duke Street, Suite 500

Alexandria, VA 22314

(800) 227-CRFA (800-227-2732)

(703) 836-4412

Fax: (703) 836-4413

www.preventcare.org

This resource provides information on cancer prevention and early detection. Resources for current patients include a therapy planner and decision-making guides.

CancerSource.com
263 Summer Street
Boston, MA 02210-11506
www.cancersource.com
"The mission of CancerSource.com is to be the most comprehensive, accurate, and personalized source of cancer information and services available" (Web site). The site provides free cancer resources to medical professionals and patients, including recent news updates and special online programming (messages boards, live chat), and information on complementary and integrative therapies. Also includes a drug database and cancer dictionary.

CancerWise™
The University of Texas M. D. Anderson Cancer Center
1515 Holcombe Blvd., Houston, TX 77030
(800) 392-1611 (USA)
(713) 792-6161
www.cancerwise.org
"CancerWise is a monthly electronic publication that contains information about the latest advancements in cancer treatment and research, support programs and activities, and cancer prevention tips, among other cancer news and information. CancerWise is produced by The University of Texas M.D. Anderson Cancer Center" (Web site). Contains featured articles and a "cancer newsline."

Cancerfacts.com
NexCure, Inc.
1725 Westlake Avenue North
Suite 300
Seattle, WA 98109
(206) 270-0225
www.cancerfacts.com
"This online resource for cancer patients, their families, and caregivers is dedicated to delivering accurate and personalized information at a time of need" (Web site). Offers cancer news

and links to local support groups. Also offers the NexProfiler™ Tool to "help people with cancer make informed treatment decisions" (Web site).

Centers for Disease Control and Prevention (CDC)
1600 Clifton Road
Atlanta, GA 30333
(800) 311-3435
(404) 639-3534
www.cdc.gov
www.cdc.gov/cancer (Cancer Prevention and Control
   Information)
The CDC's mission is "to promote health and quality of life by
   preventing and controlling disease, injury, and disability" (Web
   site). You can search for information on a wide range of medical topics, including cancer-specific issues. Much information
   is also provided in Spanish.

Gilda's Club
Gilda's Club Worldwide
322 Eighth Avenue, Suite 1402
New York, NY 10001
(888) GILDA-4-U
www.gildasclub.org
"The mission of Gilda's Club is to provide meeting places where
   men, women and children living with cancer and their families
   and friends can join with others to build emotional and social
   support as a supplement to medical care. Free of charge and a
   nonprofit, Gilda's Club offers support and networking groups,
   lectures, workshops, and social events in a nonresidential,
   homelike setting." (Web site) The organization is named after
   the comedian, Gilda Radner, who died of cancer. Call or visit
   the Web site to learn more about the support services they provide and if there is a club in your area. An online directory of
   cancer type-specific resources is available. Information on the
   Web site is offered in both English and Spanish.

Department of Veterans Affairs
Veterans Health Association
810 Vermont Avenue, NW
Washington, DC 20420
(800) 827-1000 (local VA office)

(202) 273-5400 (Washington, D.C. office)

www.va.gov

This site provides extensive information for veterans. It is a one-stop site for all concerns regarding veterans health benefits and services. Eligibility forms can be either downloaded or completed online.

CancerConsultants

411 6th Street

Ketchum, ID 83340

(208) 727-6880

www.cancerconsultants.com

"CancerConsultants is the comprehensive cancer resource. Cancer patients and their families can access the most current information about treatment, side effects, support, resources and clinical trials to facilitate informed decisions. In addition, healthy individuals can access the latest screening and prevention strategies for all types of cancer." (Web site) In addition to cancer news, this site offers a cancer dictionary and a drug dictionary.

Harvard Center for Cancer Prevention

677 Huntington Ave, Building 2, Room 105

Boston, MA 02115

(617) 432-0038

www.hsph.harvard.edu/cancer

Information and research on cancer prevention.

Health Resources and Services Administration (HRSA)

Hill-Burton Program

U.S. Department of Health and Human Services

Parklawn Building

5600 Fishers Lane

Rockville, MD 20857

(800)-638-0742

(301) 443-5656

(800) 492-0359 (if calling from the Maryland area)

www.hrsa.gov/osp/dfcr/about/aboutdiv.htm

Under the aegis of the U.S. Department of Health and Human Services, the HRSA Web site provides information on many government initiatives and programs related to providing health care to low income and disadvantaged populations.

LanguageLine Services
1 Lower Ragsdale Drive
Building 2
Monterey, CA 93940
(877) 886-3885
www.languageline.com
The "Personal Interpreter" is a "pay-as-you-go service that allows
you to access interpreters in more than 140 languages from any
phone, 24 hours a day, 7 days a week, 365 days a year." (Web
site). There is a fee to use these services if your hospital does
not have a contract with the company; you can use a credit card
to pay. The Web site also provides a description of the services
provided, including document translation.

National Cancer Institute
National Cancer Institute Public Information Office
Building 31, Room 10A31
31 Center Drive, MSC 2580
Bethesda, MD 20892-2580
(800) 4CANCER (800-422-6237): Spanish-speaking operators
available
www.nci.nih.gov and www.cancer.gov
Provides extensive information about health-related issues,
including information on cancer. The Web site includes information on how to cope with specific treatment side effects,
such as pain and fatigue, information on support and coping,
and the latest on cancer treatment and prevention. Publishes a
variety of pamphlets, including:
Chemotherapy and You: A Guide to Self-Help During Treatment
*Eating Hints for Cancer Patients Before, During, and After Treat-
ment*
Get Relief From Cancer Pain
Helping Yourself During Chemotherapy
*Questions and Answers About Pain Control: A Guide for People with
Cancer and Their Families*
*Taking Time: Support for People With Cancer and the People Who
Care About Them*
Taking Part in Clinical Trials: What Cancer Patients Need to Know
*Radiation Therapy and You: A Guide to Self-Help During Cancer
Treatment*

Available in Spanish:
* *Datos sobre el tratamiento de quimioterapia contra el cancer*
* *El tratamiento de radioterapia; guia para el paciente durante el tratamiento*
* *En que consisten los estudios clinicos? Un folleto para los pacientes de cancer*

National Center for Complementary and Alternative Medicine
NCCAM Clearinghouse
P.O. Box 7923
Gaithersburg, MD 20898
(888) 644-6226
www.nccam.nih.gov
This site provides information regarding disease-specific alternative and complementary therapies. The site covers the basics on using these therapies, where to find doctors, research, and clinical trials all related to complementary and alternative medicine. Some information available in Spanish.

National Comprehensive Cancer Network
500 Old York Road, Suite 250
Jenkintown, PA 19046
(888) 909-NCCN (888-909-6226)
www.nccn.org
This site provides information about cancer treatment centers around the U.S. It gives specific information regarding those institutions, their specialties, facilities, and resources. The site also provides cancer treatment guidelines specifically written for the patients and caregivers (approved and co-written by the American Cancer Society), such as:
Cancer Pain Treatment Guidelines for Patients
Nausea and Vomiting Treatment Guidelines for Patient with Cancer
Available in Spanish:
* *Cáncer de la próstata*
* *El dolor asociado con el cáncer*

National Coalition for Cancer Survivorship (NCCS)
1010 Wayne Avenue, Suite 770
Silver Spring, MD 20910
(877) NCCS-YES (877-622-7937)
www.canceradvocacy.org

NCCS acts as a clearinghouse for credible information about survivorship and empowers cancer survivors through its publications and programs. They publish useful pamphlets and books (see below) on many aspects of managing the medical, financial, and emotional aspects of cancer. You can order, or listen online to, the "Cancer Survivor's Toolbox" (produced in conjunction with Association of Oncology Social workers and the Oncology Nursing Society, and available in Chinese, English, and Spanish). Publishes and sells a variety of useful books and pamphlets, including:

Working It Out: Your Employment Rights As a Cancer Survivor
What Cancer Survivors Need to Know About Health Insurance
Self-Advocacy: A Cancer Survivor's Handbook
You Have The Right To Be Hopeful
Teamwork: The Cancer Patient's Guide To Talking With Your Doctor
Cancer Survival Toolbox®
A Cancer Survivor's Almanac: Charting Your Journey

National Family Caregivers Association (NFCA)
10400 Connecticut Avenue, Suite 500
Kensington, MD 20895-3944
(800) 896-3650
www.nfcarcares.org
Espousing a philosophy of self-advocacy and self-care, the NFCA provides a variety of educational materials (available through their Web site) to support family caregivers.

National Hospice and Palliative Care Organization (NHPCO)
1700 Diagonal Road, Suite 625
Alexandria, VA 22314
(800) 658-8898
www.nhpco.org
Provides information on hospice services nationally, including information on communication about hospice, insurance coverage and locating hospice services. Provides explanations of palliative care, Medicare benefits, and other frequently asked questions. Information is also available in Spanish.

NeedyMeds, Inc.
P. O. Box 63716
Philadelphia, PA 19147
(215) 625-9609
www.needymeds.com
Offers information about programs sponsored by pharmaceutical
manufacturers to help people who cannot afford to purchase
necessary drugs.

New LifeStyles Online
4144 N. Central Expressway, Suite 1000
Dallas, TX 75204
(800) 869-9549
www.newlifestyles.com
Provides information on independent retirement communities,
assisted living, nursing homes, Alzheimer's care, and home or
hospice care. You can order a free guide or search online.

Meals on Wheels
1414 Prince St., Suite 302
Alexandria, VA 22314
(703) 548-5558
www.mowaa.org
This organization provides home-delivered meals to those in
need, such as people who have trouble grocery shopping or
cooking their own food. The Web site allows you to search for
local programs.

Social Security Administration (SSA)
Office of Public Inquiries
Windsor Park Building
6401 Security Blvd.
Baltimore, MD 21235
(800) 772-1213
(800) 325-0778 (TTY)
www.ssa.gov
This Federal program provides extensive information on Social
Security Benefits including Social Security Disability (SSD),
Medicare, Supplemental Security Income (SSI), contact information to state Medicaid offices, and much more. You may be
able to apply online to these programs, and even check your

claim status. Information is available in many languages; call or check the Web site for a complete list.

The National Council on the Aging
300 D Street, SW
Suite 801
Washington, DC 20024
(202) 479-1200
(202) 479-6674 (TDD)
unitedseniorshealth.org
This is a non-profit organization focusing on informing the older consumer regarding all types of medical issues. The site provides a list of resources and publications that are specifically designed to help older individuals cope with various health issues, and offers a Benefits Checkup tool that screens seniors' eligibility for benefit programs.

United Ostomy Association, Inc. (UOA)
19772 MacArthur Boulevard, Suite 200
Irvine, CA 92612-2405
(800) 826-0826
www.uoa.org
The UOA "is a volunteer-based health organization dedicated to providing education, information, support and advocacy for people who have had or will have intestinal or urinary diversions." (Web site) Coordinates educational and support groups through local chapters, and publishes the "Ostomy Quarterly." Provides information on practical ostomy care issues, including answers to common insurance coverage questions, support information, and a Young Adult Network.

U.S. Department of Health and Human Services (HHS)
200 Independence Avenue
Washington, DC 20201
(877) 696-6775
www.hhs.gov
The mission of this government organization is to "protect health and give a special helping hand to those who need assistance." HHS provides information on many topics, including Medicare, Medicaid, childcare and health initiatives, referrals to information on cancer, and much more. HHS publishes the "Guide to Health Insurance for People with Medicare."

U.S. Department of Labor
Frances Perkins Building
200 Constitution Avenue, NW
Washington, DC 20210
(866) 4-USA-DOL
www.dol.gov/elaws/esa/fmla/fmlamenu.asp
The U.S. Department of Labor has created an online program to
help people understand their eligibility for and rights regarding
the Family Medical Leave Act. Additional information regarding employee rights, including health plans and benefits, is
available on the e-laws section of the Web site.

Post-Treatment Resource Program
Memorial Sloan-Kettering Cancer Center
215 E. 68th Street, Ground Floor
New York, NY 10021
(212) 717-3527
This organization focuses on facilitating support groups, sponsoring educational lectures, and providing other support services
to people who have completed their cancer treatment.

The Wellness Community
National Office
919 18th Street, NW
Suite 54
Washington, DC 20006
(888) 793-WELL (888-793-9355)
(202) 659-9709
www.thewellnesscommunity.org
This organization provides supportive services to people with
cancer and their loved ones by offering a variety of services,
including online information and support (through the "Virtual
Wellness Community") and on-site locations nationwide. Also
includes a list of suggested books addressing common issues
people with cancer and their families face. Information is provided in both English and Spanish.

Web Sites on Specific Topics

Bone Cancer

Osteosarcoma Online
www.iucc.iu.edu/osteosarcoma
Seeks to improve survival and quality of life for teens and young
adults with osteosarcoma through advances in patient care,
education, and research. The site is operated by the Osteosarcoma Clinical Care and Research Program, which is sponsored
by the Indiana University Cancer Center.

Breast and Gynecological Cancers

National Alliance of Breast Cancer Organizations
9 East 37th Street
10th Floor
New York City, NY 10016
(888)-80-NABCO (888-806-2226)
www.nabco.org
This organization provides information, referrals, and advocacy.
All services are free of charge. In addition to information for
people diagnosed with breast cancer, information and support
is also available for family and caregivers. On the Web site, see
the section titled "Friends & Family" for useful information
and links to additional resources intended for caregivers.

Reach to Recovery – American Cancer Society (ACS)
National Office
1599 Clifton Road, NE
Atlanta, GA 30329
(800) ACS-2345
www.cancer.org
"Reach to Recovery" is one of the many programs sponsored by
ACS providing information and support by trained volunteers
to people diagnosed with breast cancer.

**Women's Cancer Network: Gynecological Cancer Foundation
(GCF)**
401 N. Michigan Avenue
Chicago, IL 60611
(312) 644-6610

Appendix

www.wcn.org
www.wcn.org/gcf

The mission of the GCF is to "ensure public awareness of gynecologic cancer prevention, early diagnosis and proper treatment as well as support research and training related to gynecologic cancers. GCF advances this mission by increasing public and private funds that aid in the development and implementation of programs to meet these goals" (Web site). The GCF Web site contains a lot of information on the newest clinical trials, interventions to enhance quality of life, and opportunities to order educational materials. The GCF runs the Women's Cancer Network, which provides medical information, resources, and guidance for people diagnosed with gynecological cancer. The Web site incorporates topics on prevention and screening for many types of cancer, as well as inspirational survivorship stories posted on the "Wall of Hope." Articles are available in both English and Spanish.

Brain Tumors

American Brain Tumor Association (ABTA)

2720 River Road
Des Plaines, IL 60018
(800) 886-2282
www.abta.org

ABTA is an independent non-profit organization, with services including over 20 publications, addressing brain tumors, their treatment, and coping with the disease for all age groups. ABTA provides free social service consultations, a mentorship program for new brain tumor support group leaders, a nationwide database of established support groups, the "Connections" pen-pal program, networking with organizations that provide services to brain tumor patients and their families, and a resource listing of physicians offering investigative treatments. Services are offered free of charge to patients and their families.

National Brain Tumor Foundation (NBTF)

414 Thirteenth St, Suite 700
Oakland, CA 94612
(800) 934-CURE
(510) 839-9779
www.braintumor.org

"This Web site was created by brain tumor patients, family members, friends, doctors, and nurses to achieve three primary objectives: 1) Provide objective information regarding treatment options and community resources that will allow patients and family members to make decisions that best meet their own needs and values; 2) Provide a wide range of opportunities to connect with patients, caregivers, family members and healthcare providers to support each other through meaningful dialogue, either over the Internet, in person, or by telephone; and 3) Provide hope to patients, family members and friends" (Web site). If you are interested in assisting with fund-raising, read about Angel Adventure events. They also provide training for caregivers.

The Brain Tumor Society
124 Watertown St, Suite 3-H
Watertown, MA 02472
(800) 770-TBTS (800-770-8287)
www.tbts.org
"TBTS provides patient/family information and professional support through a toll-free hotline (staffed by social workers), a newsletter, and educational materials" (CancerSource.com). The Web site provides information on finding medical information, but also includes resources about locating/starting support groups and volunteer activities coordinated by the organization.

Colorectal Cancer

Colon Cancer Alliance (CCA)
175 Ninth Avenue
New York, NY 10011
(212) 627-7451
(877) 422-2030 (Toll Free Helpline)
www.ccalliance.org
Provides advocacy, information on the medical aspects of colon cancer, and support programs, such as online group support ("CCAChat") and the 'CCA Buddies Network' which "is a peer-to-peer support system that links survivors with survivors and caregivers with caregivers, for one-on-one support" (Web site). The "Resource Center" section of the Web site also has

particularly helpful information, including recommended books, helpful organizations, and much more.

Colorectal Cancer Network (CCNetwork)
P.O. Box 182
Kensington, MD 20895
www.colorectal-cancer.net
Provides a list of Web sites and organizations, with general descriptions, all related to the medical and support aspects of coping with colorectal cancer (for both patients and caregivers). Also provides other support services, including chat rooms, support information, and a list of clinical trials related to treatment of colorectal cancer.

Head & Neck Cancers

Support for People with Oral and Head and Neck Cancer (SPOHNC)
P.O. Box 53
Locust Valley, NY 11560-0053
(800) 377-0928
info@spohnc.org
www.spohnc.org
SPOHNC is a resource for information, referrals, and support, including a survivorship network; provides resources for family members; and also publishes a regular newsletter.

International Association of Laryngectomees
Jack Henslee - IAL Executive Director
Box 691060
Stockton, CA 95269-1060
(866) IAL-FORU (866-425-3678)
ialhq@larynxlink.com
www.larynxlink.com/Main/ial.htm
This non-profit organization assists laryngectomees during the rehabilitation process. They provide information for the 250 local "Lost Chord" or "New Voice" clubs and provide information to laryngectomees, their family members, healthcare professionals, and the public toward improvement in laryngectomy programs.

Leukemia and Lymphoma

The Leukemia & Lymphoma Society
1311 Mamaroneck Avenue
White Plains, NY 10605
(800) 955-4LSA (800-955-4572)
infocenter@leukemia-lymphoma.org
www.leukemia-lymphoma.org
In addition to general information on the medical and psychosocial aspects of having leukemia or lymphoma, this resource also
provides limited financial assistance to qualified individuals.
Patient and family support groups are facilitated by mental
health professionals at locations across the county. Information
provided in Chinese, English, French, Portuguese, and
Spanish.

Lung Cancer

**Alliance for Lung Cancer Advocacy, Support & Education
(ALCASE)**
500 W. 8th Street, Suite 240
Vancouver, WA 98660
(800) 298-2436
(360) 696-2436
info@alcase.org
www.alcase.org
ALCASE is a non-profit organization dedicated solely to supporting and improving the quality of lives of people with lung
cancer. Information, support, and a phone buddy program
(individual patient-to-patient support) are provided. ALCASE
also maintains a geographic listing of in-person lung cancer
support groups.

American Lung Association
61 Broadway, 6th Floor
New York, NY 10006
(212)315-8700
www.lungusa.org
The oldest voluntary health organization in the U.S., fighting
against lung disease in all forms. Available to download, the
Web site has a "Lung Cancer Profiler," which is an online tool

that can provide information specific to a person's diagnosis to assist in making informed treatment decisions.

Pancreatic Cancer

The Pancreatic Cancer Action Network (PanCAN)
P.O. Box 1010
Torrance, CA 90505
(877) 2-PANCAN
information@pancan.org
www.pancan.org

This organization provides information and support to people with pancreatic cancer and their families, as well as raising money for research and participating in pubic policy advocacy initiatives. The Web site contains information specific to caregivers.

Sarcoma

Sarcoma Alliance
www.sarcomaalliance.org

The Web site for this organization provides basic education about sarcoma, guidance on where to find sarcoma centers, and deciding upon treatment. Also has information about a financial assistance fund that supports patients who are seeking a second opinion.

The Kristen Ann Carr Fund
www.sarcoma.com

The Kristen Ann Carr Fund "provides grants for cancer research and seeks to improve all aspects of cancer patient life with an emphasis on adolescents and young adults." Information about its programs are available through its Web site, including downloadable editions of the *Sarcoma Update*, a quarterly newsletter reporting on the latest advances in treatment.

Skin Cancer

Skin Cancer Foundation
245 Fifth Avenue, Suite 1403
New York, NY 10016
(800) SKIN-490 (800-754-6490)
info@skincancer.org
www.skincancer.org
This organization emphasizes the importance of prevention of
   skin cancer, but also provides useful, reliable information on
   the diagnosis and treatment aspects of different types of skin
   cancers.

Bone Marrow Transplant

Blood & Marrow Transplant Information Network
2900 Skokie Valley Road, Suite B
Highland Park, IL 60035
(847) 433-3313
help@bmtnews.org
www.bmtnews.org
A blood and bone marrow transplant information network which
   publishes a quarterly newsletter in addition to books relating to
   transplants. The Web site also has a list of support services
   such as a patient-to-patient volunteer network they have
   organized, as well as links to numerous other resources.

National Bone Marrow Transplant Link (BMT Link)
20411 W. 12 Mile Road, Suite 108
Southfield, MI 48076
(800) LINK-BMT (800-546-5268)
www.nbmtlink.org
"The nbmtLink is a non-profit organization specifically serving
   bone marrow/stem cell transplant (BMT) patients, their caregivers, families, and health professionals," whose mission is "to
   help patients, as well as their caregivers, families and the health
   care community meet the many challenges of bone marrow/
   stem cell transplant by providing vital information and support
   services. These services include a volunteer peer support program, resource referrals for patients and health professionals,
   and educational booklets, including: *Caregivers' Guide for Bone
   Marrow/Stem Cell Transplant: Practical Perspectives.*

National Marrow Donor Program (NMDP)
3001 Broadway Street, N.E., Suite 500
Minneapolis, MN 55413
(800) MARROW2 (800-627-7692)
www.marrow.org
The NMDP is a nonprofit organization that facilitates life-saving
blood stem cell transplants for patients who do not have a
donor in their family. Managing "the world's largest registry of
volunteer stem cell donors and cord blood units" (as stated on
their Web site), they are "working to increase access to trans-
plantation through research, advocacy, and public and professional education." Information available in Chinese, English,
Japanese, Korean, Spanish and Vietnamese.

Urological Cancers (Prostate, Renal, Bladder, Penis, and Others)

American Foundation for Urologic Disease
American Foundation for Urologic Disease, Inc.
1000 Corporate Boulevard, Suite 410
Linthicum, MD 21090
(800) 828-7866
www.afud.org
Not cancer specific, but is a charitable organization supporting
research, education, and patient advocacy "for the prevention,
detection, management, and cure of urologic disease" (Web
site) in general. There are also links through their main Web
site to other online sites devoted solely to impotence and
incontinence.

The American Urological Association, Inc.
1000 Corporate Boulevard
Linthicum, MD 21090
(866) RING AUA (866-746-4282)
www.auanet.org
AUA is a professional organization with the mission to "promote
the highest standards of urological clinical care through education, research and in the formulation of health care policy"

(Web site). This Web site includes a section called "Patient Info" providing information on urologic disorders and diseases (including cancers), referral information to doctors/specialists, and a glossary of useful medical terminology.

Bladder Cancer WebCafe

www.blcwebcafe.org

This Web site provides information on medical and psychosocial issues related to bladder cancer, including helpful practical advice about negotiating the medical system, finding the right doctor and making treatment decisions. The Web site is coordinated by a cancer survivor, Wendy Sheridan, and includes many personal stories and message boards about how people have lived with and survived bladder cancer and treatment effects.

Kidney Cancer Association (KCA)

1234 Sherman Avenue, Suite 203
Evanston, IL 60202
(800) 850-9132
www.nkca.org

This resource provides medical information intended for professionals and the public. The Web site features many links to topics such as teleconferences, treatment and prevention of kidney cancer, and the latest clinical trials. You may register online or join a mailing list to receive additional information.

Us TOO International, Inc.

5003 Fairview Avenue
Downers Grove, IL 60515
(630)795-1002
(800)80-USTOO
www.ustoo.com

A prostate cancer education and support organization with over 330 support groups worldwide; visit their Web site or call the main office for further information regarding services where you live.

Alternative Therapies

American Academy of Medical Acupuncture (AAMA)
4929 Wilshire Boulevard, Suite 428
Los Angeles, CA 90010
(323) 937-5514
www.medicalacupuncture.org
Provides information on what medical acupuncture is and how it
   can be used to treat certain conditions. The Web site includes a
   list of commonly asked questions and the ability to search for
   an acupuncturist in your area.

National Center for Complementary and Alternative Medicine (NCCAM)
National Institutes of Health
Bethesda, MD 20892
(888) 644-6226
www.nccam.nih.gov
Provides an overview of what complementary and alternative
   medicine practices are, and lists clinical trials, research, news
   and events.

Chemotherapy

You are Not Alone
Post Office Box 641103
Los Angeles, CA 90064-1103
(301) 471-1766
www.yana.org
Offers online and in-person support groups for those going
   through high-dose chemotherapy. Groups currently are offered
   in California, but other in-person groups are starting in other
   areas of the United States, and online support is available.

Cancer Supportive Care
(510) 649-8177
www.cancersupportivecare.com/pharmacy.html
Drug information for chemotherapy and hormonal therapy,
   including information on financial assistance.

Clinical Trials

National Cancer Institute
(contact information located earlier in this Appendix)
www.cancer.gov/clinical_trials
CancerTrials Web site lists current clinical trials that have been reviewed by NCI. Information available in English and in Spanish.

Diet and Nutrition

Center for Nutrition Policy and Promotion (CNPP)
3101 Park Center Drive, Rm. 1034
Alexandria, VA 22302-1594
(703) 305-7600
www.usda.gov/cnpp
As part of the Department of Agriculture, this Web site provides information on general nutrition-related topics.

American Institute for Cancer Research
1759 R Street NW
Washington, DC 20009
(800) 843-8114
www.aicr.org
"AICR supports research into the role of diet and nutrition in the prevention and treatment of cancer. It also offers a wide range of cancer prevention education programs and publications for health professionals and the public. Through these pioneering efforts, AICR has helped focus attention on the link between cancer and the choices we make about food and drink, exercise, weight and smoking." (Web site) Tips on how to reduce cancer risk, including information on diet as well as menu suggestions and recipes.

Cancer Research Foundation of America's
"Healthy Eating Suggestions"
1600 Duke Street, Suite 500
Alexandria, VA 22314
(800) 227-2732
www.preventcancer.org

"The Cancer Research and Prevention Foundation, formerly the Cancer Research Foundation of America, is a national, non-profit health foundation whose mission is the prevention and early detection of cancer through scientific research and education" (Web site). You may read and order information about all types of cancer prevention, including healthy eating habits.

Fertility Resources

FertileHOPE
P.O Box 624
New York, NY 10014
www.fertilehope.org
Non-profit organization with the specific focus on providing information about cancer and fertility, such as fertility risks, fertility preservation options, the state of current research, and financial issues.

Genetic Counseling

The National Society of Genetic Counselors
Executive Office
233 Canterbury Dr.
Wallingford, PA 19086-6617
(610) 872-7608 (voicemail)
www.nsgc.org
This organization provides useful professional and consumer information. The Web site offers a feature to search for genetic counselors in your area, as well as tips on creating a comprehensive family medical history.

The National Cancer Institute (NCI)
(contact information listed earlier)
www.cancer.gov/search/genetics_services
The NCI has a searchable database on the Web site of health care professionals who specialize in genetics and can provide information and counseling.

Legal Protections, Financial Resources, and Insurance Coverage

The American Cancer Society
(contact information listed earlier)
www.cancer.org
Search using keyword "insurance." Provides information to help
   you understand your coverage and legal protections, in addition
   to how to find possible financial assistance.

Centers for Medicaid and Medicare Services
7500 Security Boulevard
Baltimore MD 21244-1850
(800) 633-4227 (toll-free)
(866) 226-1819 (TTY toll-free)
www.cms.hhs.gov
Provides extensive information and referral information on Medicaid and Medicare, including information on individual state
   plans and how to apply.

LawHelp
www.lawhelp.org
An online legal and lawyer referral service for people with low or
   moderate income. The Web site is run by a nonprofit organization based in New York City, but has information through
   partner organizations in many other states.

The Family Ties Project
www.standbyguardianship.org
This project, funded through the U.S. Department of Health and
   Human Services, maintains the above Web site which provides
   state-by-state information where standby guardianship legislation has been enacted.

Treatment Locators: Physicians and Hospitals

AIM DocFinder
State Medical Board Executive Directors
www.docboard.org
This is an online resource by a non-profit organization providing
access to a health professional licensing database.

AMA Physician Select
American Medical Association
515 N. State Street
Chicago, IL 60610
(800) 621-8335
www.ama-assn.org/aps/amahg.htm
AMA database of demographic and professional information on
individual physicians in the United States.

American Board of Medical Specialties
1007 Church Street, Suite 404
Evanston, IL 60201
(866) ASK-ABMS
(847) 491-9091
www.abms.org
Provides verification of physician qualifications and has lists of specialists. After registering on the Web site, click on the "who's certified" button and search by physician name or by specialty.

Best Hospitals Finder (U.S. News & World Report).
www.usnews.com/usnews/nycu/health/hosptl/tophosp.htm
The *U.S. News* hospital rankings are designed to assist patients in
their search for the highest level of medical care. Database is
searchable by specialty, including the top cancer hospitals.

National Cancer Institute Designated Cancer Centers
www.cancer.gov/clinicaltrials/finding/NCI-cancer-centers/map
Online directory of NCI-designated cancer centers, 58 research-
oriented U.S. institutions recognized for scientific excellence
and extensive cancer resources. Listings feature phone contact
numbers, Web site links, and a brief summary of Web site
resources.

Association of Community Cancer Centers
Cancer Centers and Member Profiles
11600 Nebel Street, Suite 201
Rockville, MD 20852
(301) 984-9496
www.accc-cancer.org/members/map.html
Geographic listing of ACCC members with contact information
and description of cancer program and services as provided by
the member institutions.

Books

How to Help Children Through a Parent's Serious Illness
McCue, Kathleen
St. Martin's Griffin, New York, 1994

*A Cancer Survivor's Almanac: Charting Your Journey, Second
Edition.*
Hoffman, Barbara, JD (Ed)
National Coalition for Cancer Survivorship
John Wiley & Sons, 1998

*The Human Side of Cancer: Living With Hope, Coping With
Uncertainty.*
Holland, Jimmie, MD and Sheldon Lewis
HarperCollins, San Francisco, 2000

*Caregiving: A Step-by-Step Resource for Caring for the Person with
Cancer at Home*
Houts, Peter and Julia Bucher
American Cancer Society, 2003

*Informed Decision (Second Edition): The Complete Book of Cancer
Diagnosis, Treatment, and Recovery*
Eyre, Harmon, Dianne Lange and Lois Morris
American Cancer Society, 2001

*Beyond Miracles: Living with Cancer: Inspirational and Practical
Advice for Patients and Their Families*
Hersh, Stephen
NTC/Contemporary Publishing, 1997

When a Parent Has Cancer: A Guide to Caring for Your Children
Harpham, Wendy S.
HarperCollins, 1997

Facing Cancer Together: How to Help Your Friend or Loved One
Brown, Pamela, with Dave Dravecky
Augsburg Fortress Publishers, 1999

When Life Becomes Precious: The Essential Guide for Patients, Loved Ones, and Friends of Those Facing Serious Illnesses
Babcock, Elise
Bantam, 1997

Handbook for Mortals: Guidance for People Facing Serious Illness.
Lynn, Joanne and Joan Harrold
Oxford University Press, 2001

Glossary

Acupuncture: Ancient Asian system of therapy that uses long, thin needles to cure disease or relieve symptoms.

Advance directive: A document in the patient's record describing his or her wishes regarding various life-sustaining interventions in the event the patient cannot communicate directly.

Alternative medicine: Healing treatment(s) used instead of mainstream, hospital-based healthcare practice.

Ambulette: Transport service for patients, usually a van that can accommodate patients in wheelchairs.

Antiangiogenesis therapy: Experimental cancer treatment that focuses on blocking growth of new blood vessels to tumors.

Anticipatory grief: Beginning to experience the loss of someone before the person actually dies.

Attending physician: Physician in charge of a hospital patient's care.

Caregiver: One who helps another person with a serious illness do what he or she ordinarily would be able to do to meet both current and future needs.

Case manager: Also called a discharge planner. Nurse or social worker who coordinates the patient's discharge from a hospital.

Chemotherapy: (Also called "chemo") Treatment of disease using chemical substances or drugs.

Clinical nurse specialist (CNS): Nurse with a master's degree who can provide patient care and education in a medical specialty.

Clinical trials: Research projects conducted by doctors to test the safety and efficacy of new drugs, therapies, or prevention strategies on patients. Also known as research protocols or clinical studies, clinical trials are scientific experiments overseen by the U.S. Food and Drug Administration which, based on the results of the trials, decides whether or not to approve the new drugs or therapies for general use.

Colostomy: Surgery to establish an artificial connection between the lumen of the colon and the skin.

Comfort care: Focuses on treating the symptoms of disease in the later stages of the disease process.

Complementary medicine or therapies: Healing treatment(s) used together with mainstream, hospital-based medical practice.

Counseling: Mental health therapy with a professionally trained therapist (*see* Social Workers).

Defense mechanism: A psychological method of protecting oneself from anxiety or high emotional distress. Denial is an example.

Denial: A defense mechanism people use to reduce their distress. Can include minimizing the significance of a stressful event, or in the extreme, denying its existence at all.

Dietitian: A professional who plans tailored diets to meet the nutritional requirements of people with special healthcare needs.

DNA (deoxyribonucleic acid): The molecular building blocks of chromosomes. They contain and control genetic information in cells, including how they divide, grow, and function.

Do not resuscitate order (DNR): Can be a component of advance directive and a living will; specifies the medical steps to be taken in the event the patient is found to be minimally responsive with minimal life signs.

Durable medical equipment (DME): Equipment such as walkers, wheelchairs, bedside commodes, or hospital beds that can be ordered from equipment suppliers for home use.

Education groups: A gathering of people where information is presented on a range of topics (i.e., coping techniques, relaxation methods, management of medical issues).

Experimental protocol: Research of a new drug or therapy using very specific materials and steps.

Fellow: Physician-in-training working in a teaching hospital.

Genetic counselor: An expert in genetics, a branch of science focused on the transmission and consequences of biologic inheritance.

Health care proxy: A document (also called medical durable power of attorney or health care agent) designating a family member, guardian, or friend as the decision-maker about medical treatment for a patient (*see* Surrogate).

Health Maintenance Organization (HMO): An organization providing health care to enrolled members through a network of member doctors and other healthcare providers. Designed to reduce costs, HMOs also typically restrict access to providers or specialists outside their approved networks.

Home care: Medical, nursing, social, or rehabilitative services provided in the patient's home.

Home health aide: Qualified person able to assist a patient with bathing, dressing, getting around in his or her own home, and doing other homemaking tasks (also, Personal care attendant).

Hospice care: Facility or home care program designed to help meet the physical and emotional needs of the terminally ill.

Hypnosis: Artificially induced trance-like state of consciousness in which the subject is susceptible to suggestion. Used in symptom relief and to reinforce behavioral change.

Incapacitated (mentally): Term used when patient is deemed by the medical team as being unable to give informed consent for a medical procedure (i.e., comatose, mentally disoriented; see Health Care Proxy).

Informed consent: After a patient is educated about his or her diagnosis and all reasonable procedures and treatments options for the disease, he or she must indicate an understanding and agreement to a course of action by signing forms.

Intern: Physician-in-training working in a teaching hospital.

Last will and testament: Legal document specifying a person's wishes with regard to inheritance after the person dies.

Licensed practical nurse (LPN): Has completed a two-year degree in nursing; often involved with hands-on patient care.

Living will: Legal document that specifies a patient's wishes in the event he or she becomes mentally incapacitated.

Living trust: A legal document created for a person while he or she is still alive in order to protect financial assets. A financial planner or lawyer can provide details.

Lumen: The area inside a hollow organ.

Malignancy: Tumors that are characterized by the ability to invade surrounding tissue and spread to other parts of the body.

Mastectomy: Surgical removal of the breast.

Medicaid: Federal- and state-funded health insurance program for those on a limited income.

Medicare: Federally run health insurance program for those aged 65 or more, on Social Security Disability, legally blind, or on renal dialysis.

Metastasis: The spread of cancer from the primary (original) tumor to another part of the body.

Nurse Practitioner (NP): Advanced practice clinician with a master's degree who can prescribe medications and write medical orders.

Nursing home: Facility that provides long-term custodial care for patients who can no longer live at home.

Nutritionist: An expert in food and drink intake (diet) for therapeutic purposes.

Oncologist: Physician expert in the treatment of cancer; includes overseeing administration of chemotherapy and other regimens.

Ostomy: Surgery to create an opening from the skin to the urinary or gastrointestinal canal, or the trachea.

Palliate: To reduce the severity of, to mitigate. Palliative care focuses on treating the symptoms of disease rather than curing it.

Paratransit programs: Local public transport system for those with a physical impairment or medical condition.

Patient confidentiality: Legal limits as to what the medical team can tell people other than the patient and his or her spouse or designated surrogate/health care proxy.

Personal Emergency Response System (PERS): Device a patient can wear that can alert emergency help.

Phobia: Overwhelming fear of an object, situation, or procedure.

Physician assistant (PA): Medical professional who can diagnose, treat and write prescriptions under a physician's guidance.

Physiatrist: A doctor who specializes in rehabilitation medicine.

Phytochemicals: Chemicals found in plants.

Positive coping: Techniques of thinking and behaving that help a patient respond to an event or stress more effectively.

Power of Attorney: A surrogate or proxy decision maker for the patient who legally makes all health-related and financial decisions for the patient; entails a legal document.

Primary caregiver: One who provides or organizes others to provide the essential logistical and emotional support for a person with cancer.

Prognosis: Prediction of the course of a disease.

Protocol: Description of a clinical trial; also used more generally to refer to a plan of medical treatment.

Progressive relaxation: Relaxation technique using deep breathing and muscle control exercises; can also incorporate peaceful music and guided imagery.

Prostatectomy: Surgical removal of part or all of the prostate.

Public assistance: Federally run program to provide cash benefits (food stamps, welfare) for persons with a low-income to purchase food and clothing and to pay for housing.

Radiation oncologist: Physician expert in radiation therapy.

Radiation therapy: Used in both diagnosis and treatment, the application of light, short radio waves, ultraviolet, or X-rays upon a specific area of the body for a period of time.

Registered Nurse (RN): Provides patient care; usually has completed a four-year college degree and hospital training.

Resident: Physician who has completed an internship and is receiving training in a specialized area.

Skilled nursing facility (SNF): A healthcare facility providing short-term nursing care with the aim of having the patient return home or to a family member's home.

Skilled nursing need: A need for services or care that can be performed only by a licensed nurse, such as treating a wound, teaching the administration of new medications, or assessing clinical status at home. Often a requirement for home care by insurers..

Social Security: Federally run program that provides monthly payments to persons over age 65 and family survivors; the amount is calculated from the person's work history.

Social Security Disability (SSD): Federally run program that provides a monthly income to disabled workers and their families.

Social Workers: Certified or licensed social workers (CSW, LCSW, LSW) usually have a master's degree (MSW, MSSW) or doctorate (DSW, PhD), and counsel the patient and family coping with the stress of diagnosis and treatment. These professionals also can identify community mental health resources and coordinate patient discharge.

Standby guardian: Legally designated person who will have custody of a patient's children in the event of their parent's death or mental incapacitation.

Staging: Systems of classifying a patient's cancer by tumor size and how far it has spread in the body.

Suicidal ideation: Thoughts or plans to commit suicide.

Supplemental Security Income (SSI): Federally run program that provides income to eligible people over age 65, legally blind or disabled, who have a low income, few assets or a limited formal work history.

Support group: A gathering that is focused on sharing experiences, providing emotional support and relieving the sense of isolation. May be led by social workers or trained cancer survivor volunteers.

Supportive care: Focused on treating the symptoms of disease in the later stages of the terminal disease process.

Surgery: Removal of a tumor, organ(s) or other objects from the body and/or repair of body parts using specific resection techniques.

Surrogate decision-maker: A person designated to make health-related decisions for that patient. The medical team addresses all health care issues for the patient directly to the surrogate.

Suppression: Trying not to think about something.

Therapy groups: Group counseling to treat a specific therapeutic issue (i.e., depression, anxiety, etc.) led by a mental health professional.

Time-out: A coping strategy of removing oneself from an emotion-producing person or situation for a short period of time.

Touch therapy: Massage or acupressure.

Veterans' benefits: Financial and/or medical care and discounted prescription drugs that may be available for U.S. veterans.

Yoga: Ancient Hindu system of philosophy that employs physical exercise and diet restrictions to control the functioning of the mind and body.

Index

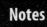

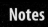